MW01283992

Case Studies in School Psychology

Case Studies in School Psychology is the first textbook to comprehensively introduce the NASP Practice Model through active discussion of real-life, school-based examples of issues facing school psychologists. Incorporating all 10 domains of practice, these true-to-life scenarios span individual child, class-wide, school-wide, and district/community-wide organizational levels across multiple age and developmental ranges. Graduate students will better understand their expansive roles and potential avenues to make positive impacts as school psychologists in children's academic, social, emotional, and behavioral development.

Stephanie A. Rahill is Associate Professor and Program Director of the School Psychology Program in the Psychology and Counseling Department at Georgian Court University, USA, and a Nationally Certified School Psychologist.

Lauren T. Kaiser is Assistant Professor and Program Coordinator of the School Psychology Program in the Psychology Department at Millersville University, USA, and a Nationally Certified School Psychologist.

Case Studies in School Psychology

Applying Standards for Professional Practice

STEPHANIE A. RAHILL
and LAUREN T. KAISER

Routledge

First published 2022
by Routledge
605 Third Avenue, New York, NY 10158

and by Routledge
2 Park Square, Milton Park, Abingdon, Oxon, OX14 4RN

Routledge is an imprint of the Taylor & Francis Group, an informa business

© 2022 Taylor & Francis

Library of Congress Cataloging-in-Publication Data
A catalog record for this book has been requested

ISBN: 978-0-367-64295-2 (hbk)
ISBN: 978-0-367-63677-7 (pbk)
ISBN: 978-1-003-12382-8 (ebk)

Typeset in Avenir and Dante
by Apex CoVantage, LLC

Contents

Tables

Figures

Acknowledgments

The list of people to acknowledge for their support in our professional endeavors, including the writing of this book, is long. First and foremost, we thank all our graduate students whom we have had the pleasure to guide towards becoming professionals in the field of school psychology. Witnessing the passion of students and their emerging motivation to become change agents in schools as they read case study examples and thought critically about the major issues within a case, was one of the major driving forces for the creation of this book. We hope that the use of a case study approach to teaching will continue to serve graduate students well in the future.

Some cases were inspired by our own children's school experiences and our experience "on the other side of the table." We acknowledge the hard work of the educators and school psychologists involved and know they are doing the best they can with what they are given. We recognize that in some cases that were used as "non-examples" there is need for support and more effective services for the staff, students, and families in the schools we serve. We acknowledge all parents out there struggling to be heard and understood as they are anxious about their own child's well-being or future. May we recognize this in all interactions and strive to join with teachers and families in problem-solving, rather than problem-admiration or -minimization. We applaud everyone's resilience despite a sometimes inadequate or flawed education system.

We recognize all our previous mentors from our training experiences. These many mentors throughout our professional lives provided of us with both the knowledge, skills, and feedback needed to thrive as professionals and the opportunities for some of the cases in this book. There are too many inspiring mentors to list, but a few we would be remiss to omit are Drs. Sylvia Rosenfield, Edward Gickling, Todd Gravois, Catherine Bradshaw, Elise Pas, and Daniel Newman. We particularly appreciate the lessons we have been taught about implementing and researching evidence-based interventions so that we could develop our vision of what works in schools. We value all of our previous faculty and acknowledge how our training incorporated the broad range of practice of school psychology that allowed us to create this case study book across all of the NASP domains of practice.

Many thanks to our own doctoral program at University of Maryland for bringing us together many moons ago as graduate students and the NASP annual conference for fostering ongoing reasons to room together year after year to continue our personal and professional bonding. Conversations about this book started at an NASP conference! We are thankful to each other for the extra push and case ideas to make it happen. Our friendship forged through the field of school psychology is a testament to the importance of having a professional collaborative relationship with someone you can also call a dear friend.

A few of the cases were inspired by the excellent work of our students in consultation, practicum, or internship cases. Notably, thank you to Shelby Grubesky and Katie Fritz for sharing parts of their work in schools as inspiration for case development. A huge thank you goes to Sara Kahan who was instrumental in assisting us with some of the detail work and logistics for this book and leading the way in setting up graphs of our example data in excel.

Thank you to friends who served as sounding boards about the writing of this book, as well as a host of other "life" issues. The daily walks during the pandemic with Debbie and Rosemary for Stephanie and daily phone calls with Denise for Lauren were a saving grace and needed self-care breaks day after day.

Last, but certainly not least, we need to recognize the support our families, mostly for not interrupting our Zoom collaborative writing calls too much during COVID-19 remote work and schooling! Thanks for giving us the space to work to Mike, Ian, Brandon, and Alec Rahill as well as Ryan, Tailiyah, Kaijiri, James, and William Kaiser. Thank you also to our parents, Charles and Lorraine Bauer and Arthur and Mary Costas, for supporting all our educational and professional endeavors throughout the years.

Introduction: A Case Study Approach to Exploring School Psychology Domains of Practice

The *Model for Comprehensive and Integrated School Psychological Services*, recently updated by the National Association of School Psychologists, provides standards for training and credentialing of future school psychologists, principles for professional ethics, and domains of practice for school psychologists (NASP, 2020). This book utilizes a case study approach to be used in training and discussion of the updated NASP Practice Model domains and Principles of Professional Ethics (PPE). The book was inspired by an educational psychology case study textbook (Ormrod & McGuire, 2007) that the first author utilized in teaching an undergraduate educational psychology course to engage students and deepen conceptual understanding. An analogous book was not available in our field of school psychology, which left us wanting as graduate educators in school psychology. Similar books are available in specific subspecialties of school psychology like consultation (e.g., Miranda, 2016; Rosenfield, 2012) or behavioral interventions (Axelrod et al., 2020), but to our knowledge, none existed for all the diverse and multifaceted aspects of our comprehensive role.

This case study approach can be used throughout a school psychology program in multiple courses where skills are introduced or deepened. A case study approach can also be utilized as part of practicum and internship classes, as school psychology candidates reflect upon their own experiences in the schools while analyzing cases. Finally, practitioners can use this case study approach to contribute to their continuing professional development. Using this case study approach, this book, or any of the individual case studies, can be used as a training tool in school psychology graduate programs and/or in-service training.

Text Structure and Connection to the NASP Practice Model

Organization of Chapters

The *Professional Standards of the National Association of School Psychologists* (NASP, 2020) provides the roadmap for our profession via the 10 domains of practice and six organizational principles, referred to as the NASP Practice Model. The NASP Practice Model is depicted as a circle (see Figure 0.1) to reflect the interrelated and interactional nature of the domains. School psychologists do not engage in specific domains of practice in isolation; rather, the work is multidimensional and requires knowledge and skills in several interrelated areas. Similarly, the organizational factors of the school and community affect the practice of school psychology.

This book utilizes the NASP Practice Model (NASP, 2020) as the organizational structure and as a training tool for developing knowledge and skills related to each domain and the organizational principles. The chapters are organized by the domains, with each chapter providing four cases to illustrate each domain. The NASP domains include: *Data-Based Decision-Making* (Domain 1), *Consultation and Collaboration* (Domain 2), *Academic Interventions and Instructional Supports* (Domain 3), *Mental and Behavioral Health Services and Interventions* (Domain 4), *School-Wide Practices to Promote Learning* (Domain 5), *Services to Promote Safe and Supportive Schools* (Domain 6), *Family, School, and Community Collaboration* (Domain 7), *Equitable Practices for Diverse Student Populations* (Domain 8), *Research and Evidence-Based Practice* (Domain 9), *Legal, Ethical, and Professional Practice* (Domain 10).

The Practice Model (NASP, 2020) also displays six organizational conditions that must be met to support effective school psychology service delivery. These principles are woven into the discussion questions and activities for each case. The organizational principles are reflective of practices within K-12 school organizations that provide the support needed for school psychologists to be effective in their roles. These organizational principles impact all areas of practice and can be considered the contextual influences on how school psychologists serve children. The organizational principles can support or hinder the work of a school psychologist, so they are important areas for analysis and reflection. The NASP's organizational principles are as

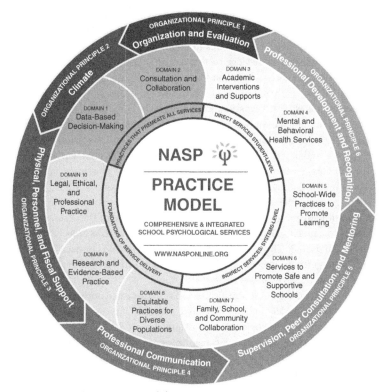

Figure 0.1 NASP Practice Model (2020)

Source: *The Professional Standards of the National Association of School Psychologists* (p. 3), by the National Association of School Psychologists, 2020 (www.nasponline.org/x55315.xml); Copyright 2020 by the National Association of School Psychologists

follows: *Organization and Evaluation of Service Delivery* (Principle 1), *Climate* (Principle 2), *Physical, Personnel, and Fiscal Support Systems* (Principle 3), *Professional Communication* (Principle 4), *Supervision, Peer Consultation, and Mentoring* (Principle 5), *Professional Development and Recognition Systems* (Principle 6).

Organization Within Chapters

Within each chapter, there is an introduction and description of that NASP domain and its importance for the practice of school psychology. Next, there is a presentation of four cases for analysis and review. Within each chapter, the cases range in complexity level from more simplistic and introductory level cases that serve to introduce the topic area to more complex cases requiring in-depth processing and prior knowledge of readers. The specific cases can be selected for discussion and analysis based on specific course level and course objectives.

After each case, there is a list of discussion questions, as well as advanced application ideas. The discussion questions are designed to inspire discussion and understanding about best practices related to the issues presented in the case. The use of discussion questions and/or advanced application questions can be selected based on whether the goal of the specific course is awareness of concepts (i.e., Introduction to School Psychology) or a more advanced-level course targeting a specific development of a set of skills (i.e., Consultation, Assessment). Some of the advanced applications allow for applied practice for advanced skills or further inquiry. In several of the cases, we refer directly to a specific chapter within the NASP *Best Practices in School Psychology* series (Harrison & Thomas, 2014) for readers to read and connect. These are merely suggestions. Readers and instructors are encouraged to make connections to other sources as well.

In the spirit of the NASP Practice Model's circular interconnections, cases do not just specifically deal with one domain of practice. Often in school psychology, the issues represent multiple domains of practice, as defined by NASP (2020). While the structure of this book categorizes cases by domains, the practice of school psychology does not occur in this type of linear fashion. Therefore, both the discussion questions and advanced applications include a notation (D1, D2, etc.) as a code for the domain(s) of practice (NASP, 2020) which might be relevant to consider when answering that question. Similarly, some of the discussion questions and advanced applications will be related to NASP's organizational principles. Those questions will be coded as follows: O1, O2, O3, O4, O5, O6.

Distinctive Case Study Features

The decision to utilize a case study approach reflects the need within graduate training to utilize real-life examples of issues that commonly occur within schools. Student exam performance and perception of their learning are increased when a case study approach is used as compared to other more traditional approaches such as textbook reading and class participation (e.g., Bonney, 2015). Critical thinking and student engagement are also enhanced using a case study approach, as well as deeper connections and integration of content (Yadav et al., 2006). Use of case studies in class may also increase class attendance (Hoag et al., 2005). While this practice needs further research to fully understand the effects of its application (Lundeberg & Yadav, 2006), particularly in the field of school psychology, it is a promising approach. We believe case discussions can lead to a deeper and richer understanding of best practices within school psychology, while engaging in ethical decision-making and incorporating research. This allows school psychologists to consider how to best serve children and their families in the school setting under challenging circumstances and barriers.

Authenticity

Each of the cases used within this book was inspired by real situations that one of the authors encountered in their practice as school psychologists or trainers. Cases were changed significantly to highlight specific practices or points of view to preserve the anonymity of people involved in the original case. Cases were also changed so they would not be recognizable, but still preserved the critical themes or features. All data associated with the cases has been altered while maintaining the central trend of data points.

Variety

The cases were selected to highlight a range of practices. In some cases, the reader will find examples of professionals utilizing best practices. In other cases, problematic behaviors of professionals working with the schools are highlighted to provide opportunities for rich discussion about the need for change and reflective practice of school psychologists. The goal of presenting cases highlighting a range of responses of various professionals is to allow readers to reflect upon how a specific case outcome, or the way a child is viewed, can be affected by various choices made by professionals working with a child. This allows the opportunity to view situations from a social justice lens and ecological perspective. The cases also allow opportunities to reflect upon the skills, values, and biases of the school psychologist and other professionals working with children, as well as the various systems-level issues in K-12 schools.

Diversity

The cases utilized in this book were selected with intentionality to represent a wide range of equity issues and developmental levels. To that end, there will be cases representing practice at all developmental levels (K to 12th grade).

The cases were also selected with the goal of representing the wide range of diverse students that school psychologists serve throughout the United States. The cases should lend themselves to open discussions around equity issues surrounding race, class, gender, culture, and ability. Cases also represent different types of difficulties that affect a child's academic, social, emotional, and behavioral progress in schools and associated contextual factors. It was not possible to include cases for all situations that a school psychologist may encounter. The cases were selected with mindfulness about the need to reflect on the broad types of school environments and situations that may occur in schools.

In selecting cases, we attempted to provide a wide range of authentic cases reflecting our years of experience in schools. However, we acknowledge that cases may be presented from our worldview and perspective as two White American middle-class women. While we continually engage in reflective practices to understand our own privileges and biases, we also understand that some of these cases may be viewed differently by others. The omission of certain cases also likely exposes our biases.

We also realize that our own blind spots as authors may be shared by many school psychology trainees, due to the ongoing concern of the lack of diversity within the field of school psychology. There is a continued need to increase diversity within our field of school psychology. According to the latest NASP membership survey (Walcott & Hyson, 2018), the field continues to be predominantly White and female. In fact, Watson and Hyson's survey results demonstrated that 88 percent of the NASP members surveyed identified as White and 83 percent identified as female. This represents an opportunity for critical analysis and to push forward the discussions within the field needed to engage with diverse populations in our schools. The open dialogue and conversations about worldview will hopefully allow for ongoing reflection of our own biases and beliefs that may impact decision-making in our work with children and families in K-12 schools. We encourage open critical analysis of the cases presented as well as discussion about the representation of diverse populations within and across cases.

One area for critical discourse may also be in the terminology used to describe the people in each case study. We acknowledge that there are diverse perspectives about identity language. We aimed to use bias-free language according to the APA bias-free language guidelines (APA, 2020), but know that individual differences exist in terms of preferences for terminology. For example, in some cases, we may use the term *Latinx* to describe a student. We used that term because it is the most inclusive of gender and ethnic origin. Using an inclusive cultural term may be the most respectful, while allowing us to preserve cultural aspects of the case and without identifying the original specific ethnic origin of the person in the case. Similarly, we used person-first language throughout the text (e.g., person with autism), but recognize that some individuals prefer identity-first language (e.g., autistic person). Discussion about preferred and respectful identity language is an important part of school psychology training. We hope these cases lend themselves well to those discussions.

How to Use This Book to Leverage Learning

We hope that this book is a helpful learning tool in your classrooms as it has been in ours. The following includes some suggested ways to maximize use of this text. This includes the description of possible approaches for utilizing case studies to enhance instructional outcomes. It also includes support for selecting cases for specific course purposes.

Case Study Approach to Teaching

To produce the positive student learning outcomes described previously, there are multiple ways to use this text to apply a case study approach within school psychology training. In his review of the literature on case study teaching, Herreid (2011) describes the multiple methods of case study use in instruction including: lectures, "clickers," discussion, individual cases, and small-group cases. These different approaches require different time commitments and may yield different outcomes, with the individual and small-group case analysis producing the best learning outcomes. If time and pacing is a concern, these cases may be easily integrated into lectures in a "story-teller" approach to provide information in context of examples and non-examples. To increase opportunities to respond in larger classes, with limited time, multiple-choice questions could be created to correspond with the case for basic recall using an every-pupil-response system (e.g., "clicker" system, response cards). With a bit more time allotment, instructors may use a whole-class discussion of the cases using a debate style or Socratic seminar (for more on this strategy, see ILA / NCTE, 2020). To deepen the case study learning opportunities, more time may need to be dedicated in or out of class for individual or small-group case analysis.

For individual-level assessment or practice, students could be assigned a case as homework and asked to provide a written-response to the case study discussion questions or take one "Advanced Application" question and expand that as a project (e.g., "Research an intervention that you would recommend given the case study assessment data, develop an intervention script and fidelity measure."). The more technologically savvy school psychology trainer could develop the cases into computer simulation activities. Finally, the deepest level of training with the best hypothesized learning outcomes would be small group discussion where students teach one another and engage in cooperative learning. Students could be divided into small groups of students and each analyze the same case given the discussion questions or one of the advanced application questions. Assigning a recorder, reporter, fact finder, and time keeper would help provide a role and accountability for each member. The reporter from each group could share the highlights of their group's discussion with the larger group for whole-group discussion and instructor feedback. Alternatively, each chapter has four cases, so each group could get a different case and then present their case to the whole class to cover more case examples in a shorter time period. The interested reader should explore more on the variations of case study uses in training or assessment (e.g., Herreid, 2011).

Case Selection

As noted earlier, the book is organized by the domains of the NASP Practice Model, but these domains are closely interrelated so cases may connect well with other domains/chapters as well. As a trainer of an introduction to school psychology course, it might make the most sense to assign a chapter when you are discussing that domain (e.g., Week 8: The School Psychologist's Role in Academic Intervention and Instructional Supports, read Chapter 3, Domain 3) and utilize those cases for class discussion that week. However, for trainers of a skill or domain specific course, it may be best to pick and choose related cases from each of the chapters. All 40 of the cases could be used in an introduction to school psychology, general practicum, or internship course. Many or all the cases can also be used in a systems-level course to analyze the organizational principles that may be operating in the individual case. The discussion questions and advanced applications labeled with a letter "O" are ripe for systems-level analysis. For planning which cases to use in a more specific skill-focused course, Table 0.1 provides a list of skills and topics within each case for trainers interested in selecting cases for specific courses or skills.

With the wide variety of opportunities to utilize the cases within this book, we anticipate that you will be able to make connections between the range of

Table 0.1 Case Skills and Topics for Selection in Specialized Courses

Domain/Case Title	Specific Skill/Topic Area	Course Types
Domain 1 Case 1 *Inequities Unearthed*	-Race/equity issues -Individual and systems-level consultation -School/family collaboration -Math CBM; math instruction & intervention -Accommodations vs specialized instruction	-Social Justice -Consultation -Academic Assessment & Intervention -Ethics and Law
Domain 1 Case 2 *A Tale of Two Classes*	-MTSS, reading -Individual and systems-level consultation -School climate assessment -Universal screening, reading	-Consultation -Academic Assessment & Intervention
Domain 1 Case 3 *A Long Wait for Assistance*	-Gender bias, academic achievement -Family collaboration -Writing assessment and intervention -Problem-solving -ADHD, inattention, motivation -Special education eligibility (OHI)	-Social Justice -Consultation -Academic Assessment & Intervention -Mental Health/ Behavior Assessment & Intervention -Ethics and Law
Domain 1 Case 4 *Understanding Cassie's Concerns*	-Assessment: socio-emotional, behavior rating, cognitive -Integrated report writing -Special education eligibility (ED/OHI) -Providing assessment results	-Cognitive Assessment -Mental Health/ Behavior Assessment & Intervention -Ethics and Law -Family/School Collaboration

(Continued)

Table 0.1 (continued)

Domain/Case Title	Specific Skill/Topic Area	Course Types
Domain 2 Case 1 *Making the Match*	-Instructional Consultation -Disproportionality and nondiscriminatory assessment of English learners -Instructional Assessment, reading -Evidence-based reading interventions -Intervention fidelity -Special education eligibility (ID)	-Social Justice -Consultation -Cognitive Assessment -Academic Assessment & Intervention -Ethics and Law
Domain 2 Case 2 *Giving Psychology Away*	-Multicultural Consultation -Instructional Assessment, reading -Reading comprehension intervention -Reading progress monitoring, CBM	-Academic Assessment & Intervention -Consultation
Domain 2 Case 3 *Reframing Resistance*	-Culturally responsive teacher coaching model -Teacher implicit bias -Teacher praise -Class ecology observation -Positive Behavior Intervention Supports	-Consultation -Mental Health/ Behavior Assessment & Intervention
Domain 2 Case 4 *Parent Consultation in the Era of COVID-19*	-Family collaboration -Academic progress monitoring, CBM -Behavioral observation methods, virtual -Behavioral interventions for online engagement	-Consultation -Academic Assessment & Intervention -Mental Health/ Behavior Assessment & Intervention

Domain 3 Case 1 *Math Skill by Treatment Interaction*	-Math CBM -Math intervention -Problem-solving teams	-Academic Assessment & Intervention -Consultation
Domain 3 Case 2 *Preempting Pre-Referral*	-Instructional Consultation -Teacher 'resistance' -Writing CBA/CBM and intervention -Special education eligibility (SLD-Writing) -Problem-solving teams	-Consultation -Academic Assessment & Intervention -Ethics and Law
Domain 3 Case 3 *Pitfalls & Plateaus*	-Instructional Consultation -Problem-solving teams -Reading CBA & interventions -Intervention fidelity -Nondiscriminatory assessment: EL students	-Consultation -Academic Assessment & Intervention -Social Justice -Ethics and Law
Domain 3 Case 4 *Dystaughtia*	-Problem-solving teams -Norm-referenced academic assessment -Grade versus age scores -Reading interventions -Special education eligibility (SLD) -IEP goals and services	-Cognitive Assessment -Academic Assessment & Intervention -Ethics and Law -Social Justice

(Continued)

Table 0.1 (continued)

Domain/Case Title	Specific Skill/Topic Area	Course Types
Domain 4 Case 1 *Screening for Intervention*	-School-wide climate data -School discipline -Social Emotional Intervention -Perceptions of aggression -Culturally responsive practice	-Systems-level Change -Mental Health/Behavior Assessment & Intervention -Counseling/Group Counseling -Social Justice
Domain 4 Case 2 *Mounting Pressures*	-Counseling -Adolescent concerns -Transition to college -Discipline vs. mental health support	-Counseling -Mental Health/Behavior Assessment & Intervention
Domain 4 Case 3 *Class-wide Intervention*	-Class-wide behavior intervention planning -Consultation -Problem-solving/Intervention design -Professional issues	-Consultation -Mental Health/Behavior Assessment & Intervention -Systems-level Change
Domain 4 Case 4 *When the Pandemic Came Along*	-Response to pandemic -Tele-health -Parent/school collaboration -Student motivation vs. mental health concerns -Child isolation	-Consultation -Mental Health/Behavior Assessment & Intervention -Ethics and Law -Counseling

Domain 5 Case 1 *Beyond Token Rewards*	-PBIS -School-wide implementation of programs -Professional development -Intervention acceptability & fidelity -Disproportionate discipline by race/ethnicity	-Systems-level Change -Social Justice -Consultation -Mental Health/Behavior Assessment & Intervention -Ethics and Law
Domain 5 Case 2 *Comparing Standard Protocol and Problem-Solving Approaches*	-Standard protocol vs. problem-solving approaches -MTSS -Science of Reading -School-wide intervention -Consultation	-Systems-level Change -Consultation -Academic Assessment & Intervention
Domain 5 Case 3 *School Diversity Climate Assessment and Intervention*	-Race/ethnicity and SES -Cultural mismatches -Affinity groups -Family/school/community collaboration -School Climate Survey Data	-Systems-level Change -Social Justice -Ethics and Law
Domain 5 Case 4 *Prioritizing Time with Fellow School Psychologists*	-Professional development -Community building -Needs assessment/Survey design -School psychology mentoring	-Ethics and Law -Professional Issues/School Psychology

(Continued)

Table 0.1 (continued)

Domain/Case Title	Specific Skill/Topic Area	Course Types
Domain 6 Case 1 *A Once-in-A-Lifetime Storm*	-Crisis response, natural disasters, short & long term -Trauma-informed care	-School Crisis Prevention and Intervention -Systems-level Change -Mental Health Assessment & Intervention -Counseling
Domain 6 Case 2 *An Ill-Advised Promise of Confidentiality*	-Suicide prevention and intervention -Confidentiality -Crisis intervention and response -Counseling ethics	-School Crisis Prevention and Intervention -Ethics and Law -Counseling -Ethics & Law
Domain 6 Case 3 *Threat Assessment Gone Wrong?*	-Threat assessment -Community engagement and partnerships with law enforcement -Problem-solving and team decision-making -School/family collaboration -Zero tolerance policies	-School Crisis Prevention and Intervention -Systems-Level Change -Ethics and Law -Counseling -Consultation
Domain 6 Case 4 *A Climate of Bullying*	-School-wide climate surveys -Bullying/aggression -School safety	- School Crisis Prevention and Intervention -Systems-level Change -Ethics and Law

Domain 7 Case 1 *Fostering Relationships*	-Foster children -Trauma-informed care -Social Justice -Academic progress and intervention -Academic intervention design (Math) -School/family collaboration -FBA/BIP	-Social Justice -Academic Assessment and Intervention -Mental Health/Behavior Assessment & Intervention -Ethics and Law
Domain 7 Case 2 *Language Differences or Deficits?*	-Social justice/academic equity issues -Working effectively with EL families -Staff perceptions and cultural mismatches -Cross-cultural competency -Family/school engagement strategies	-Social Justice Ethics and Law -Systems-level Change
Domain 7 Case 3 *Expanding the School's Knowledge Base*	-Low-incidence disabilities: Visual-impairment -Family engagement/collaboration - Community agency partnerships -Professional Development -IEP development: visual-impairments	-Ethics and Law -School/family collaboration -Professional Issues/School Psychology
Domain 7 Case 4 *Who is this Report Written for Anyway?*	-Report-writing -Team functioning -Family/school collaboration -IEP/Eligibility meetings	-Cognitive Assessment -Academic Assessment -Mental Health/Behavioral Assessment -Ethics and Law

(Continued)

Table 0.1 (continued)

Domain/Case Title	Specific Skill/Topic Area	Course Types
Domain 8 Case 1 *Digging into Discipline Data*	-Disproportionate discipline -PBIS Teams -Implicit biases, equity -Data-based decision-making -Consultation/collaboration	-Social Justice -Ethics and Law -Systems-level Change -Consultation
Domain 8 Case 2 *Zero Tolerance*	-Prevention of youth violence and substance use -Response to gang activity -School engagement for at-risk children -Multicultural Counseling -Threat Assessment	-Social Justice -Counseling -Systems-level Change -Ethics and Law
Domain 8 Case 3 *Unacclaimed and Under-represented*	-Equity in gifted identification -Universal screening -Data-based decision-making -Methods of gifted identification	-Social Justice -Cognitive Assessment -Academic Assessment & Intervention -Systems-level Change
Domain 8 Case 4 *Transition*	-Transgender youth -Supporting parents of transgender youth -Professional development	-Social Justice -Systems-level Change -Mental Health/Behavior Assessment & Intervention

	Topics	Domains
Domain 9 Case 1 *The Case for Effective Instruction*	-School psychologists as consumers of research -Analyzing special education referral patterns -Dyslexia/learning disabilities in reading -Effective Tier I instruction -Science of Reading	-Research Methods -Academic Assessment & Intervention -Systems-level Change
Domain 9 Case 2 *Evaluating Intervention Integrity*	-MTSS -Intervention acceptability & integrity -Implementation Science	-Research Methods -Consultation -Systems-level Change
Domain 9 Case 3 *The Time Crunch*	-School-wide depression screening -Analysis of assessment instruments -Cornerstones of measurement - Intervention planning -Norm groups applicability	-Research Methods -Ethics and Law -Mental Health/Behavioral Assessment & Intervention -Systems-level Change
Domain 9 Case 4 *Evaluating School-Wide Programs*	-Restorative practices -Student misbehavior/discipline -Implementation science -Program evaluation -Zero tolerance policies	-Research Methods -Systems-level Change -Mental Health/Behavioral Assessment & Intervention
Domain 10 Case 1 *Colleague Indiscretions*	-Professional issues -Ethical decision-making -Collaboration with administrators -School psychologist evaluations -Social power differences -School-wide climate	-Ethics and Law -Professional Issues/School Psychology

(Continued)

Table 0.1 (continued)

Domain/Case Title	Specific Skill/Topic Area	Course Types
Domain 10 Case 2 *Idle Gossip vs. Professional Information*	- Confidentiality -Child advocacy -Counseling -Family/School collaboration -Social media ethics	-Ethics and Law -Counseling -Professional Issues/School Psychology
Domain 10 Case 3 *Jack of All Trades?*	-Rural school psychology practice -Ethics/providing services outside of expertise -Eating disorders -Family/school/community collaboration	-Ethics and Law -Counseling -Mental Health/Behavioral Assessment & Intervention
Domain 10 Case 4 *Applying Law to Practice*	-Student chronic illness (leukemia), academic impact -504 plans (eligibility) - Family/school/community collaboration	-Ethics and Law Counseling -Academic Assessment & Intervention

experiences that school psychologists have within the schools and the NASP Practice Model. We hope that you will find the case study approach helpful to your training experience.

References

American Psychological Association. (2020). *Bias-free language.* https://apastyle.apa.org/style-grammar-guidelines/bias-free-language

Axelrod, M. I., Coolong-Chaffin, M., & Hawkins, R. O. (2020). *School-based behavioral intervention case studies: Effective problem-solving for school psychologists.* Routledge.

Bonney, K. M. (2015). Case study teaching method improves student performance and perceptions of learning gains. *Journal of Microbiology Education, 16*(1), 21–28.

Harrison, P., & Thomas, T. (Eds.). (2014). *Best practices in school psychology.* National Association of School Psychology.

Herreid, C. F. (2011). Case study teaching. In C. M. Wehlburg (Ed.), *New directions for teaching and learning, no. 128* (pp. 31–40). Wiley Periodicals, Inc. doi:10.1002/tl.466

Hoag, K. A., Lillie, J. K., & Hoppe, R. (2005). Piloting case-based instruction in a didactic clinical immunology course. *Clinical Laboratory Science, 18*(4), 213–220.

International Literacy Association/National Council Teachers of English. (2020). *Strategy guide Socratic seminars.* Read Write Think. www.readwritethink.org/professional-development/strategy-guides/socratic-seminars-30600.html#research-basis

Lundeberg, M., & Yadav, A. (2006). Assessment of case study teaching: Where do we go from here? Part I. *Jounral of College Science Teaching, 35*(6), 8–13.

Miranda, A. (2016). *Consultation across cultural contexts: Consultee-centered case studies.* Routledge.

National Association of School Psychology. (2020). *The Professional Standards of the National Association of School Psychologists.* National Association of School Psychologists.

Ormrod, J. E., & McGuire, D. J. (2007). *Case studies: Applying educational psychology* (2nd ed.). Pearson.

Rosenfield, S. A. (2012). *Becoming a school consultant: Lessons learned.* Routledge.

Walcott, C. M., & Hyson, D. (2018). *Results from the NASP 2015 membership survey, part one: Demographics and employment conditions* [Research report]. National Association of School Psychologists.

Yadav, A., Lundeberg, M. A., Dirkin, K., Schiller, N., & Herreid, C. F. (2006). *National survey of faculty perceptions of case-based instruction in science.* Paper presented at the annual meeting of American Educational Research Association, San Francisco, CA.

School Psychologists as Data-Based Decision Makers

1

Domain 1: Data-Based Decision-Making

"School psychologists understand and utilize assessment methods for identifying strengths and needs; developing effective interventions, services, and programs; and measuring progress and outcomes within a multitiered system of supports. School psychologists use a problem-solving framework as the basis for all professional activities. School psychologists systematically collect data from multiple sources as a foundation for decision-making at the individual, group, and systems levels, and they consider ecological factors (e.g., classroom, family, and community characteristics) as a context for assessment and intervention"(NASP, 2020, p. 3).

An essential skill for school psychologists is the ability to collect, understand, and analyze different types of data for the purposes of decision-making for individual students, classes, schools, and districts. This critical skill includes the ability to collect and analyze data from multiple sources to understand the needs of students. According to NASP (2020), data should be collected and analyzed for the purposes of making instructional, mental health and behavioral intervention decisions and to develop appropriate evidence-based interventions related to academic and/or behavioral needs. Further, data collection and analysis at the school or systems-level is imperative to understand so that school teams and various stakeholders can understand areas for systems-level improvement to better support all students. The ability to analyze data to determine potential inequities in instruction or access to intervention is also needed at the class-wide and school-wide level to allow for continual improvement in processes to ensure positive outcomes for all students. The first two cases highlight data-based decision-making at the systems level. In Case One, "Inequities Unearthed," the focus is on how statewide academic data can be used to understand potential inequities that a school needs to address in a systematic, structural manner. The second case, "A Tale of Two Classes" provides an example of how schools might use data to make decisions when using a multitiered systems of support (MTSS) framework.

School psychologists also utilize data to design and monitor intervention plans for students. Data should be collected to monitor and analyze intervention fidelity and acceptability. Progress monitoring, including using technological resources to collect and graph data, can be a key contribution of school psychologists while working with interdisciplinary teams, teachers, and parents to support student development. Finally, school psychologists with their advanced understanding of data collection and analysis can work to ensure that valid and reliable data collection procedures are utilized throughout all school processes (NASP, 2020). Collecting and analyzing data from multiple sources who might have varying viewpoints is the key aspect of Case Three, "A Long Wait for Assistance." This case brings the focus of data analysis to the individual student level as a team tries to understand a high school student's academic and behavioral struggles. The final case in this chapter, "Understanding Cassie's Concerns," presents cognitive, academic, and social/emotional data for a child referred for a special education evaluation.

Overall, the cases in this chapter highlight some of the different types of data that school psychologists might be tasked with analyzing for the purpose of making decisions to benefit students, teachers, and schools. The range of cases presented allows for analyses of different types of data, from an individual to a systems level, and encourages ongoing discussion of how to utilize data for decision-making in schools. In two of the cases, the issue of differing levels of concern between parents and school personnel is highlighted. In essence, there are differing views of the problem. This allows for opportunity to discuss how to better communicate and establish effective working alliances between families and schools. It also allows for reflection on how data can help inform decision-making. Further, since different stakeholders may be using different sources of data to form opinions, this highlights the importance of the school psychologist's role in collecting and reviewing multiple sources of data to help resolve conflicts.

Case One: Inequities Unearthed

At a recent IEP meeting at Abacus Middle School, a parent expressed her concerns about her son's lack of progress in math. Malcolm, a Black sixth-grade student with an IEP for an "other health impairment" for attention deficit hyperactivity disorder (ADHD) was earning decent grades from the teachers' perspective, so the teachers were not concerned with his academic progress. They tried to reassure his mother that "Cs are good grades" and that "he's in the average range and right where he should be." His mother wasn't upset about the grades per se, but she was concerned because despite his decent overall grade in math class, he was still failing every major unit assessment. She also noticed that, on his fall benchmark assessment score report that came in the mail, he scored slightly below the 10th percentile. She felt that the assessments were a sign that he was not mastering the skills that he would need to do well in math in the future. She worked with Malcolm on math at home and could see that he still had trouble answering basic math facts accurately and quickly, often still using his fingers to count. He also struggled with computation such as adding fractions with unlike denominators and long division. Additionally, math was the class in which Malcolm had the most behavioral concerns.

The teacher sent several emails and notes home about his disruptive behavior in that class. Therefore, his mom had a sense that her son likely was misbehaving to distract from having to do work that was too hard for him. The teachers disagreed and felt that he was capable of the work, especially because he was permitted to use a calculator, if he had difficulty. Visibly frustrated, Malcolm's mother was adamant in asking the team what they were going to do differently to try to help her son gain the basic skills he would need so that he would not have to overly rely on a calculator. She did not want an accommodation. Rather, his mother wanted an intervention to be utilized that would help him improve his basic math skills. The team pushed back because they said the math teachers do not have time for basic computation in their rigorous curriculum. The team said the only way Malcolm could get that help would be to give up an elective and take an extra period of math intervention. His mother was reluctant to pull her child out of an art or music class because he also really benefitted from having a break in his day as well as exposure to the arts. Listening to all of this, the school psychologist, Ms. Marzetti could see the dilemma from both sides, but was not sure how to interject.

Later, after school, Ms. Marzetti was curious to see if this was a problem for just the student or if perhaps the parent was on to a bigger issue. The annual state math assessment data was available on the state's website for each school, so Ms. Marzetti decided to take a closer look. After reviewing the school level data (see Table 1.1), Ms. Marzetti's concerns grew. She could see immediate issues with equity in both math and English language arts (ELA), especially for Black, Latinx, English learners, students with disabilities, and economically disadvantaged students. Committed to doing something about this, Ms. Marzetti approached the math teacher after the meeting to offer consultative services. Specifically, Ms. Marzetti conducted three two-minute division computation skills curriculum-based measurement (CBM) probes with Malcolm. Malcolm's median score was 15, which was at a frustration level for the student and below the 25th percentile. The teachers were not willing to alter their instruction for new intervention ideas, so Ms. Marzetti offered to provide Malcolm direct services for 15 minutes per day during his math period. She worked with the student using a very simple strategy of timed fluency practice interspersing easy and hard

Table 1.1 Sixth-Grade Math State Assessment Data for Abacus Middle School

	Percent Proficient	
	Math	ELA
Asian	92%	85%
Black/African American	21%	37%
Hispanic/Latino	39%	45%
White	70%	75%
Two or More Races	50%	62%
Students With Disabilities	13%	10%
English Learner	38%	35%
Economically Disadvantaged	12%	25%
ALL	**65%**	**70%**

math problems (Hawkins et al., 2005; Intervention Central, n.d.) to keep his motivation high. Calculating his accuracy and observing his daily practice, she was able to see some of his errors and help provide brief error correction and targeted explicit instruction in the skill he needed (e.g., long division with a zero in the quotient). Within just a few weeks, Malcolm made considerable progress towards instructional and mastery level. She graphed his progress in order to share with the team and parent at the next meeting (see Figure 1.1).

Discussion Questions

1. What type of data did the school psychologist, Ms. Marzetti, use to make decisions in this case? How did that data influence the case outcomes? (**D1**)
2. What other interpretations would you make when looking at these data? What other questions or concerns do these data raise? (**D1, D8**)
3. What are the implications of the school's perspective that the child's grades of C are not a problem? What does this potentially mean regarding the expectations set for this specific child? (**D1, D8**)
4. What other data might have been helpful for the team to consider in this case? (**D1**)
5. While Ms. Marzetti used data to make decisions, it sounded like she did this in isolation of the team or math teacher and provided direct service. How might she have approached this differently from a consultative perspective? What might have happened had she approached it with indirect services? (**D2, O4**)
6. Ms. Marzetti offered direct services for an individual student. While this had positive outcomes for the student, what about the other group equity issues she observed in the data? How might she have approached this same data from a school-wide systems service delivery perspective? (**D5**)
7. It sounded as if the parent was feeling frustrated and alone in the IEP meeting, from a family-school collaboration perspective, what could the team and Ms. Marzetti have done differently? (**D7**)
8. The IEP Team and parent seem to have a difference of perspective on the role of the IEP in terms of emphasizing accommodations or specialized instruction. What is the difference between the two? What purposes do they each serve? Why should the team consider both accommodations and specialized instruction to support this student? (**D10**)

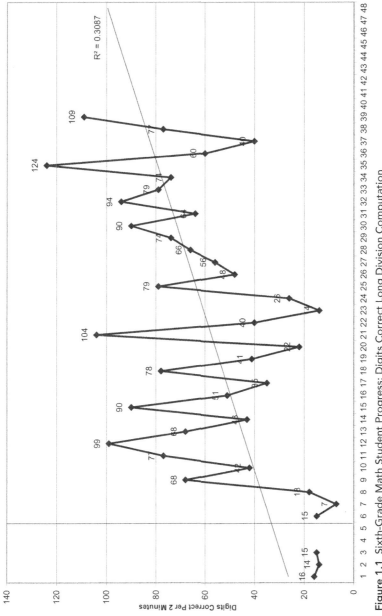

Figure 1.1 Sixth-Grade Math Student Progress: Digits Correct Long Division Computation

Advanced Applications

1. Role-play this team meeting with classmates in groups of at least four (roles: parent, math teacher, school psychologist, process observer). The teacher and parent can play their role as described in the scenario. The school psychologist should attempt to take a more active role in the meeting, using collaborative and reflective communication skills to create a shared understanding of the concerns and help the parent and teacher work more effectively towards solutions. The observer should take notes on the communication skills used to give positive and constructive feedback. **(D2, D7)**

2. The teacher in this case expressed concerns embedding computation strategies into their curriculum. How might you work with them to suggest a class-wide intervention like the individual intervention Ms. Marzetti used individually with the student in this case? Review universal math intervention protocols (e.g., VanDerHeyden, 2020) to develop an intervention script, treatment fidelity and progress monitoring plan. **(D3)**

3. Examine similar school-level data for a school in your area (e.g., the school where you shadowed a school psychologist; a practicum site; etc.). Search public websites (e.g., school, district, state) to see what public data exist (e.g., state assessment data, climate surveys) and if the data are aggregated by groups. View the data with an eye for equity issues. Share these data with your class to discuss, generate hypotheses, and plans for additional data that would be helpful to collect for problem-solving purposes. **(D1, D8)**

4. In her best practices chapter, Habedank Stewart (2014) discusses best practices in the development of academic local norms. After reviewing this discussion of how a school or school district might go about creating local norms, apply a strategy to this case. How could the school develop local norms for math skills that could be helpful in ensuring that students received extra instruction when needed, regardless of their grades in a specific math class? Create a plan for the development of these norms. **(D1)**

Case Two: A Tale of Two Classes

The school psychologist, Dr. James, at Henry Hudson Elementary School is a key member of the school's MTSS team. The school is a small K-4 school with two classes per grade. One of the team's responsibilities is the academic screening of all children in the elementary school. The school completes a reading screening for all students three times per year (Fall, Winter, and Spring) and students receive tiered instruction based on the results of the reading screening measures. At this particular school, students at the Tier II level receive small group targeted reading intervention/instruction three times per week. Students at the Tier III level receive individual instruction in the resource room twice per week in addition to the small group instruction. It is now February and the team has become concerned with the number of students who are either referred for special education evaluation or who are receiving intensive services at the Tier III level. The academic interventionists who are working with students in Tier III are reporting that they are getting overwhelmed with the number of children who they are working with at this level. They report feeling frustrated that so many students are placed in Tier III and they do not believe that there are adequate systems in place to ensure high quality Tier I and Tier II instruction. This has led to some negative interactions amongst the staff with some staff feeling like they are carrying the bulk of the workload for other teachers.

The school psychologist, Dr. James, is tasked with reviewing the data to determine trends and assist with decision-making based on the data. Upon reviewing the data for the two second-grade classrooms in the school, Dr. James finds the following trends in data:

- In one second-grade classroom, 94 percent of students are making adequate progress with Tier I Instruction, 3 percent of students are receiving targeted Tier II supports, and 3 percent are receiving intensive Tier III interventions.
- In the other second-grade classroom, only 30 percent of students are making adequate progress with Tier I Instruction. Sixty percent of students are receiving Tier II targeted supports, and 10 percent are receiving intensive Tier III interventions.

Dr. James initially wonders whether the students had been assigned to their class based upon previous academic performance, which had been a practice of the school in the past. However, the administrative team confirms that a random assignment occurred the previous summer to ensure heterogeneous groupings in the second-grade classrooms.

Discussion Questions

1. What hypotheses should Dr. James and the MTSS team consider when analyzing this data from the second-grade classrooms? What might be going on here? (**D1**)

2.   What should the school psychologist do next? What other data might be necessary to understand student performance? (**D1**)

3.   Should Dr. James and the team decide to conduct some classroom observations in the two second-grade classrooms, what should be the goal of the observations? What should they be observing in the classroom environment specifically? (**D1**)

4.   How might Dr. James and/or the team potentially provide consultation with one of these teachers? How might the possibility of consultation be approached? (**D2**)

5.   If there are concerns that there are behavior management and difficulties with effective instruction at the Tier I level in the one second-grade classroom, what should Dr. James do next? Is this an administrative issue that should be reported? What are the ethical implications of the next steps taken? (**D10, O1**)

6.   The case refers to some negative interactions between staff members. Why might this be the case? Why should Dr. James and the principal be concerned with the negative feelings that might occur among staff members regarding workload? (**O2, O4**)

Advanced Applications

1.   Research the elements that should be included in effective Tier I instruction. How can MTSS teams determine whether those elements are in place in their schools? What if they were not in place? (**D3, D4**)

2.   Dr. James realizes that they have not been collecting data on intervention integrity. Research some guidelines for how the team might proceed in developing an intervention integrity process for Tier I, Tier II, and Tier III interventions. (**D1**)

3.   Based on your decisions on types of classroom observations needed in discussion question number three, design an observation protocol for use in classes to observe Tier I instruction. (**D1**)

4.   What strategies might be needed to improve the school climate at this school? (**O2**)

Case Three: A Long Wait for Assistance

Leslie is a White, ninth-grade student who has been referred to the Child Study Team by her English teacher at the high school. According to this teacher's referral, Leslie does not attend to what is going on in the classroom. She doesn't seem to pay attention in class and often falls asleep in class. Leslie's teacher is concerned that Leslie has poor motivation and believes that this may be due to an underlying mental health issue that should be addressed. The teacher also suggests that perhaps Leslie should be evaluated for Attention Deficit Hyperactivity Disorder (ADHD), primarily the inattentive type, due to her difficulties with attending to the class lectures and producing assignments in a timely manner. This English teacher also emphasizes that Leslie is a well-liked teenager who has wonderful social and prosocial communication skills. She indicates that Leslie is the first to greet the teacher every morning with a bright, sunny smile and a big hello. She also reports that Leslie seems to be well liked by her classmates. However, once class starts, the teacher almost immediately begins to see Leslie's sunny disposition disappear. She will slump in her chair with her shoulders down and stare out the window during instructions. The teacher has also noticed Leslie's classmates offering her assistance with writing assignments.

As part of the pre-referral process, the team solicits input from all of Leslie's teachers. The reports returned from teachers indicate that she rarely turns in any homework, particularly in her English and History classes. Both of those teachers indicate that the quality of the work that she does submit is typically poor. It is also reported by those teachers that she completes in-class written assignments at an extremely slow rate. In fact, when asked to write during class, this is often when she will fall asleep. She is currently failing both History and English. She has a D in Biology, and grades of A in Math, Band, and Art. The Biology teacher reported that while she is very engaged and does quite well on all the in-class laboratory assignments; he is concerned that Leslie often does not write-up the lab results in the required lab reports. If she does submit the written lab reports, they are poorly written and lack the required details. He indicated that she seems to understand the lab and can understand complex research questions, but for some reason does not follow through in displaying this understanding in her lab write-ups.

A Child Study Team meeting is held with Leslie's mother in attendance to discuss possible avenues for intervention for Leslie. In the meeting, Leslie's mother indicated great relief that "finally a school is seeing that there is a problem here." Leslie's mother reported that Leslie has struggled with reading comprehension and writing throughout her elementary and middle school years. However, when she would bring this up to teachers in parent-teacher conferences, she was often told that Leslie was progressing just fine, that she was only a little below grade level in reading and writing skills and that she was an absolute pleasure to have in class. Leslie's mother firmly believes that Leslie's pleasant personality and advanced communication skills led to teachers in elementary/middle school dismissing problem areas. She cries during the meeting at the prospect of getting some assistance academically for Leslie. She reported that Leslie used to spend hours in elementary school and middle school on her homework assignments, often leading to tears and frustration. Leslie's mother has also noticed that since beginning high school, Leslie does not seem to have a lot of homework. When told that Leslie has not turned in many homework assignments, Leslie's mother was surprised. She expressed worry that Leslie is now just "giving up on school."

Discussion Questions

1. What hypotheses should the Child Study Team explore to better understand Leslie's performance in various classes? (**D1**)
2. What additional data does the Child Study Team need to assist in understanding some of the concerns that have been presented about Leslie's academic performance? (**D1**)
3. How might the difference between Leslie's grades in different high school classes be explained? (**D1**)
4. Leslie's mother expresses that her concerns as a parent were dismissed throughout Leslie's schooling. What are some potential issues with the parent-school relationship that occurred and what could have/should have been done differently earlier in Leslie's schooling? (**D7**)
5. Should any data collection that might occur next include an evaluation for ADHD? Why or why not? (**D1**)
6. How might the fact that Leslie is a female have impacted on the decisions that have been made throughout her schooling regarding her need for additional support/services? How about the fact that she is White? Could this have played a role in decision-making? Why or why not? (**D8**)
7. Discuss how Leslie's positive pro-social skills may have masked academic concerns throughout her schooling. Could her academic deficits have been overlooked because she presents as competent socially? (**D4**)
8. What should be the next step for the Child Study Team? Is an evaluation for special education services warranted? Why or why not? (**D1**)

Advanced Applications

1. Research motivation in children. What do we know about motivation and the connections between motivation and academic performance?

Given what the research tells us about motivation, what hypotheses might we draw about why Leslie appears unmotivated to her English teacher? (**D3, D4**)

2. Leslie's mother reports that Leslie used to spend hours completing homework in elementary school, which was a frustrating and exhausting process. Research best practices for homework assignments. How much homework should be assigned based on developmental level? What type of homework assignments are appropriate for various classes and developmental levels? (**D3**)

3. It appears that many of the academic concerns that were reported by Leslie's mother throughout her schooling were dismissed. What systems or structures should be in place in schools to ensure that all students receive the academic, social, emotional, and behavioral supports they need to be successful? What type of system could have been of assistance to Leslie throughout her elementary and middle school years? Why? (**D5**)

Case Four: Understanding Cassie's Concerns

Cassie is a 9-year-old, third-grade White student who initially was referred for an evaluation due to concerns with emotional difficulties as well as academic difficulties. The Child Study Team agreed that a full evaluation would be helpful due to her ongoing academic and behavioral difficulties in school. The following presents summaries of some of the evaluation data from the school psychologist's evaluation. Standardized assessment test data are presented in Tables 1.2, 1.3, and 1.4.

Cassie was referred for a psychological evaluation by her counselor and parents due to concerns regarding her current social/emotional functioning. The referral questions of interest to her parents include strategies for assisting her in becoming happier and developing a more positive self-esteem. Cassie's teacher is concerned that her academic performance is very uneven. At times, she can produce good work; however, she also will struggle with completing assignments and has a history of poor performance on quizzes and tests. Her current grades include Cs and Ds in all academic subjects, As and Bs in her elective classes (physical education, music, and art).

Cassie was generally quiet throughout evaluation sessions but responded appropriately to all tasks and questions asked of her. Hearing and gross/fine motor coordination appeared appropriate. She initially appeared uncomfortable in the testing environment and rapport with the examiner was established over an extended period. She was concerned about the length of the

Table 1.2 Standardized Assessment Data Sheet: WISC-V

Wechsler Intelligence Scale for Children-V (WISC-V)	Standard Score (95% Confidence Interval)	Percentile Rank	Descriptive Classification
FULL SCALE SCORE	103 (98–108)	58th	Average
VERBALCOMPREHENSION	106 (99–112)	66th	Average
Similarities	Scaled Score: 12		
Vocabulary	Scaled Score: 13		
VISUAL SPATIAL	104 (96–111)	61st	Average
Block Design	Scaled Score: 10		
Visual Puzzles	Scaled Score: 10		
FLUID REASONING	104 (96–111)	61st	Average
Matrix Reasoning	Scaled Score: 12		
Figure Weights	Scaled Score: 10		
WORKING MEMORY	104 (96–111)	61st	Average
Digit Span	Scaled Score: 10		
Picture Span	Scaled Score: 12		
PROCESSING SPEED	88 (80–98)	21st	Low Average
Coding	Scaled Score: 7		
Symbol Search	Scaled Score: 9		

testing and the amount of time that she was missing from her classes. During the testing sessions, Cassie was cooperative and appeared motivated to do well on test items. She appeared to give her best effort on all test items. She was attentive and focused throughout the sessions and demonstrated adequate levels of engagement in the testing process.

However, it was noted that when items on tests became more difficult for Cassie, she seemed to become agitated and nervous, which may have impacted her test performance. She would frequently provide explanations about why she did not know the answer. For example, she made statements such as, "This is not something we have learned yet in third grade" and "I haven't learned this yet." Cassie continued to seem worried that she

Table 1.3 Standardized Assessment Data Sheet: WJ-IV Tests of Achievement

Woodcock-Johnson IV Tests of Achievement (WJ-IV; Form A)	Standard Score	Confidence Interval (95%)	Percentile Rank	Descriptive Classification
BROAD ACHIEVEMENT	*100*	*96–103*	*49*	*Average*
Letter-Word Identification	100	93–106	50	Average
Applied Problems	103	93–113	59	Average
Spelling	95	88–102	37	Average
Passage Comprehension	106	95–117	66	Average
Calculation	96	88–104	39	Average
Writing Samples	108	98–104	39	Average
Sentence Reading Fluency	99	91–108	48	Average
Math Facts Fluency	100	91–109	50	Average
Sentence Writing Fluency	94	82–106	34	Average
BROAD READING	*101*	*94–108*	*53*	*Average*
Letter-Word Identification	100	93–106	50	Average
Passage Comprehension	106	95–117	66	Average
Sentence Reading Fluency	99	91–108	48	Average
BROAD MATHEMATICS	*100*	*94–105*	*49*	*Average*
Applied Problems	103	93–113	59	Average
Calculation	96	88–104	39	Average
Math Facts Fluency	100	91–109	50	Average

(*Continued*)

Table 1.3 (continued)

Woodcock-Johnson IV Tests of Achievement (WJ-IV; Form A)	Standard Score	Confidence Interval (95%)	Percentile Rank	Descriptive Classification
BROAD WRITTEN LANGUAGE	*98*	*93–104*	*46*	*Average*
Spelling	95	88–102	36	Average
Writing Samples	108	98–117	69	Average
Sentence Writing Fluency	94	82–106	34	Average
ACADEMIC SKILLS	*97*	*92–101*	*41*	*Average*
Letter-Word Identification	100	93–106	50	Average
Spelling	95	88–102	37	Average
Calculation	96	88–104	39	Average
ACADEMIC APPLICATIONS	*107*	*100–115*	*69*	*Average*
Applied Problems	103	93–113	59	Average
Passage Comprehension	106	95–117	66	Average
Writing Samples	108	98–117	69	Average
ACADEMIC FLUENCY	*98*	*92–104*	*46*	*Average*
Sentence Reading Fluency	99	91–108	48	Average
Math Facts Fluency	100	91–109	50	Average
Sentence Writing Fluency	94	82–106	34	Average

Table 1.4 Standardized Assessment Data Sheets: Social/Emotional and Behavioral Assessment Data

Behavior Assessment System for Children-III	Parent's Report	Teacher's Report
Composites:		
Externalizing Problems	44	48
Internalizing Problems	57	57
Behavioral Symptoms Index	61	56
Adaptive Skills	37	32
School Problems	–	56
Scales:		
Hyperactivity	50	55
Aggression	43	43
Conduct Problems	42	46
Anxiety	70	55
Depression	58	60
Somatization	39	52
Atypicality	60	59
Withdrawal	75	49
Attention Problems	53	69
Adaptability	38	37
Social Skills	50	40
Leadership	44	44
Activities of Daily Living	48	–
Functional Communication	39	56
Learning Problems	–	51
Study Skills	–	

BASC-III Self-Report	Cassie's Report (T-Scores)
Composites:	
School Problems	46
Internalizing Problems	70
Inattention/Hyperactivity	67
Emotional Symptoms Index	74
Personal Adjustment	41

(*Continued*)

Table 1.4 (continued)

BASC-III Self-Report	Cassie's Report (T-Scores)
Scales:	
Attitude to School	47
Attitude to Teachers	58
Atypicality	68
Locus of Control	55
Social Stress	75
Anxiety	75
Depression	66
Sense of Inadequacy	68
Attention Problems	70
Hyperactivity	60
Relations with Parents	63
Interpersonal Relations	36
Self-Esteem	37
Self-Reliance	38

Revised Children's Manifest Anxiety Scale (RCMAS-2)	Cassie's Self-Report (T-Scores)
Total Anxiety Scale	>80
Physiological Anxiety	71
Worry	73
Social Anxiety	>80

Children's Depression Inventory-2	Cassie's Self-Report (T-Scores)
Total Score	69
Negative Mood	59
Interpersonal Problems	71
Ineffectiveness	82
Anhedonia	58
Negative Self-Esteem	73

was not doing well with the testing, despite frequent reassurances from the examiner. At other times, she made statements such as "I'm sure other third graders can do this" and "Would you send someone back to second grade because of these tests?" providing further evidence of a high degree of anxiety revolving around the test taking process. At one point during the testing, she indicated that she was too nervous to finish the test. She commented, "I don't think that I can do the rest. I'm too nervous" and she then put her head down on the table. At this point, testing was discontinued for the day and completed the following week. When she returned for an evaluation session the following week, she was attentive and motivated and completed the assessment without further incident.

In a student interview, Cassie noted that she "frequently feels like crying," that she is "often discouraged," and that she "very frequently feels sad and gloomy." She also reported that she believed that her peers could do better than she could academically. She reported that she does not believe that she can keep up with her peers in academics, and therefore, "there is no point in trying." She reported that she often gets mad at herself when she cannot do something. This tendency was also noted in the Sentence Completion Test. For one item, she responded that, "the worst thing about me is . . . that I get really mad at myself and call myself names."

Cassie's third-grade teacher reports that Cassie has the academic skills to be successful in school. However, she often does not complete both in class and homework assignments. The teacher does not understand why she will not complete work that she clearly has the aptitude to complete. At times, Cassie seems to just "shut down" and does not engage with either the teacher or peers in the classroom. The teacher cannot identify a reason for the times when Cassie just "refuses to do the work." She also has a history of poor performance on quizzes and tests. For example, Cassie will complete the spelling homework successfully all week. However, when it comes time for the weekly spelling test on Friday, Cassie looks angry or upset before the test begins and then typically does poorly on the test. The teacher noticed her crying during the test a few times. When she approaches her to ask what is wrong, Cassie does not respond and seems embarrassed that her emotions are being pointed out by the teacher.

Discussion Questions

1. In analyzing the data presented, what are Cassie's strengths? Areas of concern? How do you know this? (Use data to support your response). (**D1**)

2. Based on your state's eligibility guidelines, do you believe that Cassie qualifies for special education services? If yes, in what category (categories)? What evidence do you have to justify qualification (or not) for special education services? **(D1, D10)**
3. Beyond decisions for special education eligibility, what types of supports do you believe that the school should put into place to support Cassie? **(D3, D4)**
4. What recommendations might be made to Cassie's parents? What types of community-based or family-based supports might be helpful? **(D7)**
5. What additional data might be needed to better understand the stated referral questions? **(D1)**

Advanced Applications

1. Organize the data presented into "themes." Use the integrated report writing worksheet presented in Table 1.5 (Rahill, 2014) to present themes and the data that supports each theme. Create additional columns (themes) as necessary.
2. In small groups, role play how you would present the findings from this evaluation to Cassie's parents. **(D2, D7)**

Table 1.5 Integrated Report Writing Worksheet

Child-Centered Theme: (strengths/weaknesses)	Theme 1:	Theme 2:	Theme 3:	Theme 4:
Evidence from Assessments (includes formal assessments, interviews, observations, file review, etc.)	1. 2. 3. 4. 5.			
Divergent information:				
Potential explanations for divergent information:				
Follow-up Assessments Needed to understand conflicting assessment results				

3. Create a list of recommendations that you might suggest for Cassie's teachers and parents to help support her. (**D3, D4**)
4. Write a sample report based on the data provided for Cassie that is integrated and easily understandable for her family. (**D1, D7**)

References

Habedank Stewart, L. (2014). Best practices in developing academic local norms. In P. L. Harrison & A. Thomas (Eds.), *Best practices in school psychology: Foundations* (pp. 301–314). National Association of School Psychologists.

Hawkins, J., Skinner, C. H., & Oliver, R. (2005). The effects of task demands and additive interspersal ratios on fifth-grade students' mathematics accuracy. *School Psychology Review, 34*(4), 543–555. https://doi.org/10.1080/02796015.2005.12088016

Intervention Central. (n.d.). *Math computation: Increase accuracy by intermixing easy and challenging computation problems.* www.interventioncentral.org/academic-interventions/math-facts/math-computation-increase-accuracy-intermixing-easy-and-challengin

National Association of School Psychology. (2020). *The professional standards of the national association of school psychologists.* National Association of School Psychologists.

Rahill, S. (2014). Theme-based psychological reports: Towards the next generation of psychological report writing. *Trainer's Forum: Journal of the Trainers of School Psychologists, 32*(2), 10–23.

VanDerHeyden, A. (2020). *Class-wide math intervention protocol. National Association of School Psychologists.* www.nasponline.org/resources-and-publications/resources-and-podcasts/covid-19-resource-center/return-to-school/considerations-for-math-intervention-upon-the-return-to-school

School Psychologists as Consultants and Collaborators

2

Domain 2: Consultation and Collaboration

"School psychologists understand varied models and strategies of consultation and collaboration applicable to individuals, families, groups, and systems, as well as methods to promote effective implementation of services. As part of a systematic and comprehensive process of effective decision making and problem solving that permeates all aspects of service delivery, school psychologists demonstrate skills to consult, collaborate, and communicate effectively with others." (NASP, 2020, p. 4)

According to NASP (2020), school psychologists use a consultation problem-solving process to deliver their services, whether they be academic, mental or behavioral health. These services can be aimed at multiple systems and levels (e.g., student, teams, school, family, or community). In order to do this, school psychologists require effective communication and relationship-building skills, as well as cultural sensitivity to work with a diverse range of stakeholders (NASP, 2020, p. 4). Zins and Erchul (2002) define consultation as,

> School consultation is defined as a method of providing preventively oriented psychological and educational services in which consultants

and consultees form cooperative partnerships and engage in a recipro-
cal, systematic problem-solving process guided by ecobehavioral principles. The goal is to enhance and empower consultee systems, thereby
promoting students' well-being and performance.

(p. 626)

A key component of this definition is the empowerment of the consultee
systems. This indirect service delivery model is what Gutkin and Conoley
(1990) refer to as the "Paradox of School Psychology," that is, to serve children effectively school psychologists must first and foremost concentrate their
attention and professional expertise on adults" (p. 203). Case Two is titled
"Giving Psychology Away," in the spirit of this paradox, which was inspired
by earlier thinking that psychologists, to be effective must engage in "giving
it [psychology] away to those who really need it" (Miller, 1969, p. 1071). It is
an example of how the school psychologist used the Instructional Consultation (IC) process to help a teacher generalize an instructional strategy to a
whole group of students, thus providing a broader indirect effect. Teacher
resistance garners much attention in the school consultation literature (e.g.,
Butler et al., 2002) and is often miscategorized in the field. At times, "resistance" might not be due to a teacher's unwillingness to change or put forth
the time. It may be due to other reasons that require more creative solutions.

The first case, "Making the Match," also highlights Instructional Consultation (IC; Rosenfield, 1987, 2014), and specifically focuses on its application
to an English learner to increase reading proficiency. This should allow for
a rich discussion of best practices for academic intervention and assessment
of all students, but particularly bilingual students, and how school psychologists are a critical part of that collaborative problem-solving process to help
teachers, even special educators, develop cultural proficiency and the ability
to create more effective instructional matches.

Case Three, "Reframing Resistance" provides an example of a teacher
coaching model, the Double Check model (Bradshaw et al., 2018), to increase
teachers' culturally responsive practices and student engagement. The
teacher in this case appears resistant, but through this case it will become
apparent that resistance was due to other factors that a skilled consultant can
help reframe to empower the teacher to change.

The final case addresses the massive increase of support that schools need
to provide for parents/families as they engaged in virtual and/or hybrid
instruction with their children during the COVID-19 pandemic. With children
mostly learning from home, parents are thrown into the role of "teacher"
and many needed ongoing support to manage the academic, behavioral, and

instructional "home-based" environments. Providing parent consultation services; therefore, has become even more critical.

The four cases in this chapter highlight just a few examples of school psychologists involved in consultation and collaboration with teachers; however, throughout this book there will be other cases representing several NASP domains of practice in which the school psychologist uses these skills with parents, administrators, teams, and across different systems levels.

Case One: Making the Match

At the beginning of the school year, Ms. Martin, the special education teacher at City Valley Elementary School, approached the new school psychologist, Ms. Estes with concerns about her sixth-grade student Tina. Ms. Martin explained to Ms. Estes that Tina was about to graduate elementary school and move on to junior high for seventh grade. Tina was receiving special education services for a mild intellectual disability and this was a reevaluation year for her. Ms. Martin wanted to get the reevaluation process started early because she was worried that Tina would need much more supports moving to junior high. Ms. Martin feared that Tina would struggle given the fact that Tina had not made progress at all since she started in special education in second grade. According to Ms. Martin, Tina had not made any progress in reading in the past three-years, not even bumping up any guided reading levels. Tina was still at an emergent reading level (e.g., primer, Level C), after several years of attempted interventions in small group and special education in a resource room. They had tried Lindamood Phoeneme Sequencing ® (LiPS ®, WWC, 2010) and Read 180® (WWC, 2016). Ms. Martin felt this must be indicative of a more severe intellectual disability and felt that reevaluation would be needed to document those needs and the need for more intensive services in junior high. Ms. Estes, being new to the school, did not know much about Tina so asked a few more background questions to understand the situation further. She found out that Tina had moved from Puerto Rico in the second grade and was a student for whom English was a second language. Several thoughts came to Ms. Estes's mind after learning that the student was not a native English speaker and that the special education placement had happened soon after arrival to their Midwest United States school. Recognizing the need to understand how second language acquisition may explain some of the student's slower progress, Ms. Estes offered consultation services to ensure that the student's lack of progress was not due to a lack of appropriate instruction or language differences.

Ms. Martin agreed to work with Ms. Estes weekly to work through the Instructional Consultation (IC, Rosenfield, 1987, 2014) process. They conducted several Instructional Assessments (IA, Gickling et al., 2016; Gravois & Gickling, 2008) to gather more information on the student's reading skills in order to create an "instructional match." Ms. Estes explained the concept of instructional match to Ms. Martin briefly, that it was when the student was reading in text with 93–97 percent accuracy or working in drill and practice activities with 70–85 percent known material and 15–30 percent unknown/new material interspersed (Gickling et al., 2016). From the IA, they determined that the student could recognize only 54 words by sight. They prioritized word-recognition, implemented a folding-in strategy ("drill sandwich") intervention (Gickling et al., 2016) with ample repetition throughout the day and opportunities to read the target words in context via instructional level teacher-made simple stories. To increase the repetition of the folding-in strategy, Ms. Martin planned to implement the strategy with Tina in small-group daily. Additionally, she was going to train Tina's other teachers, her general education teacher and her EL teacher, to implement briefly during class transitions (e.g., lining up for lunch, switching classes). With this instructional match and high degree of distributed practice in place, Tina quadrupled her word knowledge in the intervention period and moved up three guided reading levels (see Figure 2.1).

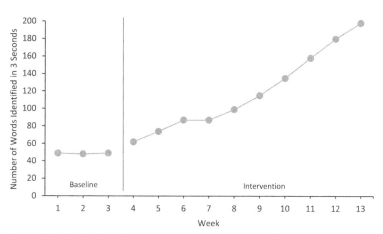

Figure 2.1 Tina's Sight Word Progress via Instructional Consultation and an Instructional Match

Discussion Questions

1. What assumptions were being made about this student by the teacher, albeit well intentioned, and how did consultation help shift those assumptions? (**D8**)
2. What do the data suggest about the student's rate of learning and response to intervention? (**D1, D3**)
3. Why might this intervention, which included high repetition throughout the day and reading texts created by the teacher with the folding-in strategy, have been more effective for Tina than the previously attempted interventions (LiPS ®, Read 180®)? (**D3, D9**)
4. What might this mean about Ms. Martin's original assumption that the student might have a more severe intellectual disability? What other data might help to make that determination? (**D1, D8, D10**)
5. What might have happened had the school psychologist proceeded with a standard cognitive assessment battery for this student without offering consultation support? (**D1, D8, D10**)

Advanced Applications

1. Review the research on the original two interventions implemented. What does the research say about those interventions? What are the advantages and disadvantages of each? (**D3, D9**)
2. Review the research on the folding-in strategy. What does the research say that intervention? What are the advantages and disadvantages? (**D3, D9**)
3. What would you suggest to Ms. Estes as an assessment battery for the formal reevaluation in terms of non-discriminatory assessment? Consult references regarding best practices in non-discriminatory assessment (Ortiz, 2014), the use of interpreters (Lopez, 2014), and assessment of English learners' literacy skills (Vanderwood & Socie, 2014). (**D1, D8, D10**)
4. In this case, intervention fidelity did not appear to be an issue, but how could Ms. Estes confirm that? Develop an intervention script and fidelity measure for the folding-in strategy. (**D1, D2, D8, D9**)

Case Two: Giving Psychology Away

Mr. Taylor is a reading teacher at Town Square Middle School, a suburban middle school. His fourth period reading intervention class is comprised of a small group of sixth-grade students, all of which are students of color. He reached out to his school psychologist, Ms. Yoshiro, for help improving the reading comprehension of one of his students, Morgan, a biracial student. As a man who identifies as biracial, Mr. Taylor felt called to ensure that he tries everything he can to help Morgan succeed. He shared with Ms. Yoshiro that he could relate to Morgan because when Mr. Taylor was in middle school, he also struggled with reading and felt marginalized in his predominantly white suburban school. Ms. Yoshiro met with Mr. Taylor to describe the IC (Rosenfield, 1987, 2014) process in greater detail to see if this was a process that he would like to commit. Mr. Taylor was interested so they set up a standing weekly meeting to work through the IC problem-solving process. Mr. Taylor was pleased with his student, Morgan's recent progress in the area of reading fluency, but noticed that although Morgan is now on-grade-level in terms of reading rate and accuracy, comprehension is still an area of concern.

Ms. Yoshiro offered to conduct an instructional assessment (IA, Gickling et al., 2016; Gravois & Gickling, 2008) with Morgan, but also with Mr. Taylor present. It was important to Ms. Yoshiro, and the IC process, that the IA be conducted collaboratively so that the teacher and her could be on the same page in terms of the observed student reading skills, but also so she could model the IA formative assessment process for Mr. Taylor. Ms. Yoshiro believes that if the teacher can learn the IA, then the teacher will be better equipped to make an instructional match for students. She offered this rationale with Mr. Taylor, who was excited to do this together and to learn a new set of assessment strategies. Through the IAs, they confirmed that Morgan's reading accuracy and fluency were not concerns. Morgan read with 99 percent accuracy and at the 50th percentile in terms or correct words read per minute. Ms. Yoshiro and Mr. Taylor prioritized reading comprehension because Morgan could answer an average of two of five comprehension questions accurately after reading a grade level passage. Their goal was to elevate comprehension question accuracy to at least four out five questions.

Ms. Yoshiro and Mr. Taylor collaboratively reviewed a few different evidence-based comprehension strategy options. Ms. Yoshiro had reviewed the research in advance in order to present the teacher with some options from which to choose. Using the elicit-provide-elicit strategy of motivational interviewing (Reinke et al., 2011), Ms. Yoshiro offered the information about all three strategies and then asked Mr. Taylor which one sounded like it would work best for the student and be the best fit in the classroom. Mr. Taylor was automatically drawn to the strategy referred to as "Forming Questions." Forming Questions is a metacognitive strategy to help students understand how questions are formed and derived from texts (Gickling et al., 2016). Recognizing the opportunity to help Mr. Taylor generalize this skill and strategy to other students, Ms. Yoshiro asked him, "are there other students in your

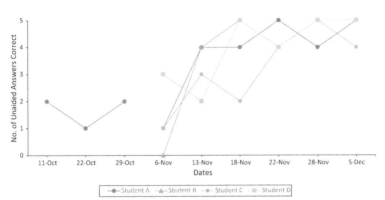

Figure 2.2 Intervention Group IC Case Progress in Reading Comprehension

class that could use this strategy?" Mt. Taylor said that his whole intervention group could really benefit from this metacognition strategy. He was eager to brainstorm a group implementation plan with Ms. Yoshiro.

They worked together to plan the details of how the strategy would be modeled for Mr. Taylor first by Ms. Yoshiro and Morgan, then Mr. Taylor would implement it together with Ms. Yoshiro and the whole group for support. After that, Mr. Taylor planned to implement the strategy on his own daily at the end of each reading lesson with his group. Mr. Taylor would then collect the reading comprehension data with all the students in that group once per week. Ms. Yoshiro and Mr. Taylor would graph that data together each week and share the progress graph with the students for motivation. They were happy to see their progress from week to week. As seen in Figure 2.2, all the students made rapid progress and met the intervention goal. Mr. Taylor expressed comfort embedding this strategy into his instruction on his own moving forward. He and Ms. Yoshiro celebrated the progress and closed their case together. Ms. Yoshiro let Mr. Taylor know that he could reach out to her again in the future if he had other concerns and wanted to work through the IC process again. He said he would gladly take her up on that offer if he has new concerns, but that he felt confident for now that he has just added a new tool to his teaching toolbox.

Discussion Questions

1. How did this school psychologist "give psychology" away in this case? (**D2, O4**)

2. NASP (2020) advocates the use of effective and appropriate interpersonal skills to serve as a change agent and lead to more provision of more effective services. What communication and collaborative skills did this school psychologist use to do this? (**D2**)
3. How might the data collection in this case have facilitated the positive teacher and student outcomes? (**D1**)
4. This diverse group of students were in a remedial reading intervention group. What might have happened to the students if the consultant and teacher did not use a problem-solving process such as this? How was this an important step in the prevention of inappropriate referrals to special education? (**D8, D10**)

Advanced Applications

1. Review the research on evidence-based reading comprehension interventions. Select three that you would propose to a teacher if you were in a similar situation as the school psychologist in this case. (**D3**)
2. In this scenario, the elicit-provide-elicit strategy (Reinke et al., 2011) was particularly helpful. In this strategy the consultant starts by asking the teacher what strategies they have in mind for the goal. Then, the consultant asks if the teacher would be interested in hearing a few other ideas. If the teacher says yes, the consultant offers the information tentatively and follows that with a question to elicit the teacher's perspective. Role-play the elicit-provide-elicit strategy using the three interventions you identified for this concern area. (**D2**)
3. What limitations are there to this data collection or graphing approach? What other data might you like to collect for this case to determine if the students are making adequate progress in reading comprehension? Pick at least one other measure and describe its advantages and limitations. (**D1**)
4. Think of this case from a multicultural consultation perspective (see Ingraham, 2000). What is the consultation constellation in this case? How might that have affected the consultation relationship? (**D8**)
5. If you were the school psychologist, what would the multicultural consultation constellation be (see Ingraham, 2000)? What might you need to do to explore your own cultural identity in relation to this case? How might you explicitly talk with Mr. Taylor about the racial aspects of the case that he raised, as well as gender? (**D8**)

Case Three: Reframing Resistance

Mr. Nash, a White male teacher, worked in a diverse urban school serving primarily low-income students. He recently made a late-career change from law enforcement to become a teacher. Ms. Mayer, the school psychologist, was recently assigned to this school and did not know many of the staff members well yet but was working to develop positive relationships in the school and offer her coaching and consultation services to anyone who was interested in problem-solving with her. She met Mr. Nash at a faculty meeting where she was taken aback by some of his negativity about the new ideas being presented by the professional developer leading the meeting. Admittedly, her first impression of him was not good. She was concerned about his toxic energy. At the same time, she often tries to give teachers the benefit of the doubt because she herself was once a teacher and knew the job can be incredibly stressful and can lead to burnout. She thought she may have just been catching him on a bad day, but in one of her first meetings with the principal of the school, she learned that the principal too was concerned with Mr. Nash's negativity.

The principal, Dr. Tamela, a Black female, confided in Ms. Mayer and shared her frustration about Mr. Nash. Dr. Tamela was concerned that the students in his class, many of whom were students of color, were being referred to the office at high rates, especially compared to the other classes. When she observed or walked by his classroom, she frequently heard him yelling or reprimanding the students. Dr. Tamela had recently placed Mr. Nash on an action plan, which is a first step in a formal process before an administrative transfer or firing. As part of the action plan, she mandated that he seek coaching to improve his teaching. The principal knew about Ms. Mayer's skills in coaching and consultation and asked her if she could coach Mr. Nash to be more culturally proficient and build stronger relationships with his students. Ms. Mayer was concerned that coaching might not be effective if it was mandated, but she offered to give it a try.

Ms. Mayer recognized that approaching Mr. Nash to offer coaching might be challenging. She delicately broached the subject by reflecting the feelings she noticed in the faculty meeting and checking in with him given that he appeared frustrated. He opened a bit to her about his frustration with his class and how the students are "the most challenging group he has ever had." She empathized with him and shared with him that Dr. Tamela told her about his action plan. She wasn't sure if that was a good idea, but felt it was best to be direct. Ms. Mayer let him know that although coaching was a mandated part of the plan, and that she was willing to be his coach, that he still had the option to say no and seek coaching from a different colleague. She informed him of the type of coaching models she had been trained in recently, one of which was a newer model called Double Check (DC, Bradshaw et al., 2018), which is a culturally responsive coaching model aimed at increasing student engagement. He liked the sound of that given that he felt his students were disengaged. Given the principal's interest in this case, Ms. Mayer realized she must address the limits of confidentiality. She reassured him that if he engaged in the process, his role would be to inform Dr. Tamela of the coaching progress. Ms. Mayer emphasized that, as his coach, she would not share any details of their coaching with Dr. Tamela, or anyone in the school, without his permission. Ms. Mayer said that she would be able to provide him with their coaching action plans and graphed data to share with the principal to indicate his participation and progress. This put him at ease, and he agreed to begin coaching.

During the initial interview phase of coaching, Mr. Nash disclosed that he is too negative with his class. He was keenly aware of the problems this caused and indicated a sincere desire to change. Mr. Nash was discouraged that he couldn't stop "eyeballing all the negative." Ms. Mayer's classroom observations and baseline data collection confirmed this. The frequency of his reprimands was significantly more than the amount of praise he provided his students, which often was limited to none. In one 10-minute observation, he reprimanded students at least 20 times, two times per minute. Ms. Mayer shared the data with him, and he recognized that if he could be more positive, and less negative, with his students it would improve their relationships and engagement. His goal was to increase his praise and decrease his reprimands. With his coach, they set a goal to reverse the praise to reprimand ratio from 1:5 to 2:1. They talked through many strategies to help him remember to praise, such as keeping a list of praise statements on a clipboard near him while he taught or keeping the school's positive behavior tokens in his pocket as a reminder to distribute them during class.

After weeks of trying to increase praise statements and decrease reprimands, with little success, Dr. Tamela approached Ms. Mayer to inquire about the case. Dr. Tamela was concerned because she was not seeing rapid changes to his teaching. Ms. Mayer was unsure how to approach this. She did not see this as Mr. Nash's resistance. She wanted to advocate for Mr. Nash, but at the same time was concerned about breaking confidentiality. She politely reminded Dr. Tamela that she could ask Mr. Nash directly to see the coaching documentation of his attempts and progress, but that she was not at liberty to break their coaching confidentiality to preserve the coaching trust they had developed. Dr. Tamela understood and respected Ms. Mayer's boundaries.

Ms. Mayer, perplexed about what to do next to help Mr. Nash reach his goal, reframed this problem from a "won't do" issue, to a "can't do" problem. In other words, she realized he may lack the skills to be more positive. She realized, after he shared with her how he only noticed the negative behaviors, that modeling was needed. It dawned on her that the students in his class were often on-task and trying to comply with his many rules, but that he just was not noticing it. Perhaps, he needed to see someone else noticing and praising all the students' positive behaviors to recognize that the students demonstrate more positive behaviors than he realized. Ms. Mayer had noticed that there was another male teacher in the school who was extremely positive with the students and highly respected in the building. She thought that perhaps Mr. Nash would fare better with a male role model than if she offered to model. With the teacher's permission, Ms. Mayer invited that teacher to co-teach a lesson with Mr. Nash. The model teacher taught the first half of the lesson while Mr. Nash and Ms. Mayer observed and collected data on the model's use of praise statements, the students' behaviors, and responses to the praise. Ms. Mayer then met with Mr. Nash to debrief the observation. Mr. Nash reflected on how many positive behaviors there were in his class that he had been missing. After allowing time to unpack that further, Mr. Nash then took over his class again with Ms. Mayer collecting data on his use of praise. He immediately increased his use of praise dramatically. After his lesson, Ms. Mayer showed him the graph (see Figure 2.3)

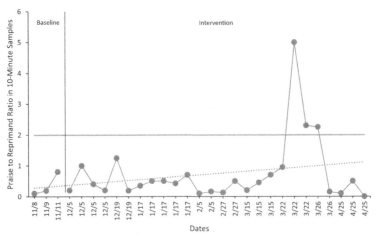

Figure 2.3 Double Check Coaching Teacher Progress Increasing Praise to Reprimand Ratio

and affirmed him for his hard work and progress. She allowed him time to reflect on how it felt and his next steps. At follow-up, praise levels decreased towards baseline again indicating the need for continued modeling/practice, but this helped confirm for Ms. Mayer that they were now on the right track.

Discussion Questions

1. What consultation and collaboration skills did this school psychologist use to enhance teacher and student outcomes? (**D2**)
2. Why was it important that the school psychologist did not view this as resistance, but from a different perspective? (**D2**)
3. What was the ethical dilemma faced by the school psychologist in this case? How did she navigate those issues? What might have happened if she handled it differently? (**D10**)
4. In the research on the efficacy of the Double Check model, Bradshaw and her colleagues (2018) found that coaches often prioritize positive behavior intervention goals but did not explicitly set cultural proficiency goals as frequently. How is that evident in this case? In this case, were the class management goals related to cultural proficiency? If yes, how? If not, what would be gained by bringing race and culture into the conversation and goals? (**D8**)

Advanced Applications

1. Review the research on methods to improve teacher praise. Based on that research, what might you suggest the coach try next if the modeling does not produce consistent increases in praise? (**D2, D4**)
2. What might the school psychologist do differently if this problem appeared to be shared by multiple teachers in the school? (**D2, D5, D6**)
3. Practice collecting observation data on teacher praise and reprimands. See the Classroom Check-Up training module for observation examples and practice (The Classroom Check-Up, 2020). (**D1**)
4. How did the collaborative culture of this school system allow for peer consultation and mentoring to occur? What would happen if the school system did not have a collaborative culture that allows for open dialogue about how to improve practices? (**O2, O5**)

Case Four: Parent Consultation in the Era of COVID-19

Sara is a school psychology intern who began her internship in Fall of 2020 during the ongoing pandemic. Luckily, Sara had completed her practicum hours during her second year of her program at the same school district, so she has some familiarity with the teachers and many of the students from her experiences the previous year. However, like many districts in her area, this school began the school year in a completely virtual environment. All students receive instruction remotely throughout the Fall and the district administration has recently announced that remote instruction will continue until at least January of 2021. With this news, Sara and the rest of the school mental health and Child Study Team professionals begin to hear more concerns from parents who are having difficulty managing their children's instruction from home. Given that many of the parents are working parents, they are reporting that they are overwhelmed with managing various academic and behavioral issues with their own work demands. Sara has begun to communicate frequently with one parent in particular, Mrs. Jackson, who is extremely concerned with her first-grade son's academic and behavioral progress and ability to manage the virtual school environment.

When Sara asks the first-grade teacher about this student, Sean, the teacher does not report any major concerns. She indicates that he seems to be progressing academically and she does not have any major concerns with how he is doing with remote learning. This is different from what Sara is hearing from his mother, Mrs. Jackson. Mrs. Jackson indicates that Sean is not able to follow along easily with what is happening virtually in the class and that it takes him hours to complete academic lessons and assignments. He struggles with managing how to open apps and other websites on the computer and needs his mother's assistance both with the logistics of managing the virtual day and with his academic assignments. His mother is extremely frustrated because she is also trying to work full-time in a virtual environment, and she is interrupted throughout the day to aid Sean. She believes that the teacher only thinks that Sean is progressing because the teacher does not see the extraordinary amount of one-to-one assistance that she must give him in order to successfully make it through his school day.

Sara would like to offer additional support to Mrs. Jackson through a parent consultation model. However, when she approaches her supervisor about this, her supervisor speaks to the teacher and then comes back to say that she does not think it is necessary because the teacher has not noted any major concerns. Sara's supervisor believes that consulting with this parent is not worthy of Sara's time, given the large caseload that they both already have. However, Sara continues to receive emails from this parent about the major concerns and decides to begin a formal consultation process with the mother. When she approaches her supervisor again about the mother's ongoing concerns, her supervisor indicates that Sara can engage in consultation with the mother but does not feel like it will do much to help.

Sara begins this process by conducting observations during the virtual environment. After the first two observations of the virtual class, Sara and Mrs. Jackson discuss the fact that Sean does seem to have difficulty following the on-screen instructions that the teacher is giving. Sara and Sean's mother collaboratively decide to focus on increasing Sean's ability to independently follow multi-step instructions from the teacher to find materials, websites, and begin independent assignments. Sara wants to collect baseline data but does not want to put this extra burden on Mrs. Jackson, given that she is already feeling overwhelmed with the demands on her during the virtual school day. Therefore, Sara devises a plan in which she can collect data herself, even though she is completing these observations in a virtual environment.

Sara conducts additional observations of the virtual environment and collects latency data, by recording how long it takes for Sean to respond to the teacher's request or instructions compared to an average peer. She records this data during both the Language Arts and Math block, which both take place in the morning. Both blocks include 30 minutes of instruction and 15 minutes of independent work time. It is noted that Sean will often turn off his camera after instructions about independent work are provided by the teacher. His mother indicates that he has learned to turn off his camera when he is going to ask his mother for assistance in finding the materials needed per the teacher's instructions. Therefore, Sara also records how many times Sean's camera is turned off during each block of instruction. See Table 2.1 and Figures 2.4 and 2.5 for Sara's depiction of the data.

In analyzing the data, Sara determines that Sean is having more difficulty than the average peer in his class, in that it takes him far longer to respond to instructions and he often turns his camera off right after instructions are given. This is presumably to go to seek out his mother's assistance, a fact that his mother confirms. Now that the problem behavior and areas of concern are defined, Sara begins the process of determining appropriate interventions that can be implemented in the home. She seeks out supervision from her supervisor at school, but the supervisor does not seem to have ideas, since working in this virtual environment is so new to her as well. Sara's supervisor tells her that she does not have any ideas or time to research the ideas. Therefore, Sara sets out to search the recent literature to determine whether she can find suitable interventions for the virtual school environment and seeks out peer supervision during her University-led internship class. Before

Table 2.1 Baseline Data for Sean and an Average Peer

	Sean	Average Peer
Baseline Day 1		
# Teacher Requests/Instructions	8	8
Mean Time in Seconds until Instruction Followed	189	83
# of Times Camera Turned off	7	1
Baseline Day 2		
# Teacher Requests/Instructions	12	12
Mean Time in Seconds until Instruction Followed	175	62
# of Times Camera Turned off	10	0
Baseline Day 3		
# Teacher Requests/Instructions	9	9
Mean Time in Seconds until Instruction Followed	211	75
# of Times Camera Turned off	9	1

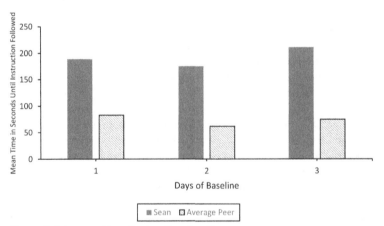

Figure 2.4 Latency Data During Baseline Phase

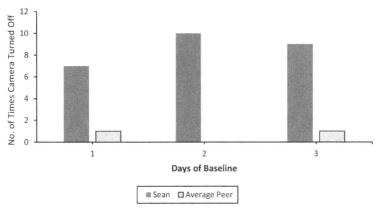

Figure 2.5 Webcam Usage During Baseline Phase

beginning to explore interventions, Sara is interested in collaborating with Mrs. Jackson to create a reasonable goal. She holds a virtual meeting with Mrs. Jackson to discuss the baseline data and collaboratively decide upon reasonable goals for Sean specifically regarding decreasing the amount of time for him to respond to teacher instructions and in needing support from his mother (measured by number of times camera is turned off).

Discussion Questions

1. Parent consultation seems to be increasingly in demand during virtual instruction and the ongoing pandemic. What are some best practices in how parent-based consultation sessions should proceed? Do you agree with Sara's decisions thus far in how she has proceeded with this parent consultation case? (**D2, D7**)

2. Sara decides to use the number of times the camera is turned off during lessons as a measure of whether Sean can follow teacher instructions. She assumes that the number of times that the camera is turned off is indicative of the number of times that he seeks assistance from his mother. Is this an accurate assumption? Although an imperfect measure, is this a reasonable measure, given the difficulties in obtaining data in virtual environments? Are there other ways that she could have obtained this information (without adding to the burden of Mrs. Jackson during home instruction)? (**D1, D7**)

3. Sara does not seem to get much supervision from her school-based internship supervisor on this case. Why might that be? How and why

might their priorities be different in this case? As the supervisor, what additional supervision would you have provided Sara? (**D10, O5**)

4. In their best practices chapter, Sullivan et al. (2014) discuss the importance of school-based supervisors understanding the research on supervision standards and practice. They also discuss the idea that interns appreciate when their supervisors are organized and deliberate in providing supervision overall and with specific cases. In what ways did Sara's supervisor not meet this expectation as a supervisor and how could this experience be improved for Sara in the future? (**D10, O5**)

Advanced Applications

1. Sara's next step is to collaboratively decide upon goals with Mrs. Jackson. What might be reasonable goals for Sean in the virtual environment? How did you arrive at this decision? (**D1, D2, D7**)

2. In looking at the data thus far, do you feel like the comparison peer also could improve upon their reaction time to teacher requests? Is it possible that a class-wide intervention by the teacher might be needed to increase understanding of instructions for all students in order to increase academic engaged time for all? (**D4, D5**)

3. Research and suggest at least interventions that could possibly be used to assist Sean in becoming more independent from his mother in proceeding through his virtual day. (**D4**)

4. Sean's academic progress has not been explicitly discussed and/or evaluation thus far in this case. Moving forward, what steps can be taken to evaluate Sean's academic performance in the virtual environment, given Mrs. Jackson's stated concerns that she does not feel like he is making adequate progress? What specific measures would you suggest and why? (**D3**)

References

Bradshaw, C. P., Pas, E. T., Bottiani, J. H., Debnam, K. J., Reinke, W. M., Herman, K. C., & Rosenberg, M. S. (2018). Promoting cultural responsivity and student engagement through Double Check coaching of classroom teachers: An efficacy study. *School Psychology Review, 47*(2), 118–134. https://doi.org/10.17105/spr-2017-0119.v47-2

Butler, T. S., Weaver, A. D., Doggett, R. A., & Watson, T. S. (2002). Countering teacher resistance in behavioral consultation: Recommendations for the school-based consultant. *The Behavior Analyst Today, 3*(3), 282–288. http://dx.doi.org/10.1037/h0099983

The Classroom Check-Up. (2020). *Procedure: Assess classroom.* www.classroomcheckup.org/coaching-process/assess-classroom/

Gickling, E. E., Gravois, T. A., & Angell, V. (2016). *Instructional assessment: An essential path for guiding reading instruction.* ICAT Publishing.

Gravois, T. A., & Gickling, E. E. (2008). Best practices in instructional assessment. In A. Thomas & J. Grimes (Eds.), *Best practices in school psychology V* (pp. 503–518). National Association of School Psychologists.

Gutkin, T. B., & Conoley, J. C. (1990). Reconceptualizing school psychology from a service delivery perspective: Implications for practice, training, and research. *Journal of School Psychology, 28*(3), 203–223. https://doi.org/10.1016/0022-4405(90)90012-V

Ingraham, C. L. (2000). Consultation through a multicultural lens: Multicultural and cross-cultural consultation in schools. *School Psychology Review, 29*(3), 320–343. https://doi.org/10.1080/02796015.2000.12086018

Lopez, E. (2014). Best practices in conducting assessments via school interpreters. In P. L. Harrison & A. Thomas (Eds.), *Best practices in school psychology: Data-based and collaborative decision making* (pp. 113–128). National Association of School Psychologists.

Miller, G. (1969). Psychology as a means of promoting human welfare. *American Psychologist, 24*(12), 1063–1075. https://doi.org/10.1037/h0028988

National Association of School Psychology. (2020). *The professional standards of the national association of school psychologists.* National Association of School Psychologists.

Ortiz, S. (2014). Best practices in nondiscriminatory assessment. In P. L. Harrison & A. Thomas (Eds.), *Best practices in school psychology: Data-based and collaborative decision making* (pp. 61–74). National Association of School Psychologists.

Reinke, W. M., Herman, K., & Sprick, R. (2011). *Motivational interviewing for effective classroom management: The Classroom Check-Up.* The Guilford Press.

Rosenfield, S. A. (1987). *Instructional consultation.* Lawrence Erlbaum Associates.

Rosenfield, S. A. (2014). Best practices in instructional consultation and instructional consultation teams. In P. L. Harrison & A. Thomas (Eds.), *Best practices in school psychology: Data-based and collaborative decision making* (pp. 509–524). National Association of School Psychologists.

Sullivan, J. R., Svenkerud, N., & Conoley, J. C. (2014). Best practices in the supervision of interns. In P. L. Harrison & A. Thomas (Eds.), *Best practices in school psychology: Foundations* (pp. 527–540). National Association of School Psychologists.

Vanderwood, M. L., & Socie, D. (2014). Best practices in assessing and improving English language learners' literacy performance. In P. L. Harrison & A. Thomas (Eds.), *Best practices in school psychology: Foundations* (pp. 89–98). National Association of School Psychologists.

What Works Clearinghouse. (2010). *WWC intervention report: Lindamood Phoneme Sequencing (LiPS®)* https://ies.ed.gov/ncee/wwc/Docs/InterventionReports/wwc_lindamood_031610.pdf

What Works Clearinghouse. (2016). *WWC intervention report: Read 180®.* https://ies.ed.gov/ncee/wwc/Docs/InterventionReports/wwc_read180_112916.pdf

Zins, J. E., & Erchul, W. P. (2002). Best practices in school consultation. In A. Thomas & J. Grimes (Eds.), *Best practices in school psychology IV* (pp. 625–643). National Association of School Psychologists.

Providing Services in Academic Interventions and Instructional Supports

3

Domain 3: Academic Interventions and Instructional Supports

"School psychologists understand the biological, cultural, and social influences on academic skills; human learning, cognitive, and developmental processes; and evidence-based curricula and instructional strategies. School psychologists, in collaboration with others, use assessment and data collection methods to implement and evaluate services that support academic skill development in children." (NASP, 2020, p. 5)

The ability to use evidence-based academic and instructional strategies to assist children in their academic development is a critically important role of a school psychologist. School psychologists should have a thorough understanding of curriculum, pedagogical principles, and instructional design for all grade levels so that they can offer their expertise in support of academic development in all children. Since school psychologists understand the connection between academic success and the mental health, social and behavioral development of children, they are in the position of assisting students, parents, and staff in supporting academic development for the benefit of the whole child.

School psychologists assist in appropriate assessment and data-based analyses to pinpoint academic difficulties with the purpose of driving sound intervention design based on identified areas of need. When a clear under-standing of academic needs is evident, school psychologists can research and suggest specific instructional interventions that are evidence-based. School psychologists can also provide support by assisting with the monitoring of student progress. With their understanding of intervention science, school psychologists are in the unique position to guide decisions regarding assess-ment, intervention, progress monitoring, and intervention integrity and acceptability. Additionally, school psychologists have expertise in the areas of cognition and learning and can offer this expertise to ensure that instructional decisions are in line with best practices and research findings in these areas. School psychologists utilize their consultation skills to provide indirect ser-vices in academic and instructional intervention for students and to work col-laboratively with other professionals in their school-based teams.

School psychologists must also ensure that they use assessments that are both culturally responsive, appropriate, fair, and necessary to make decisions about students' responsiveness to intervention and need for further academic support through special education services. The over-arching goal of assess-ment procedures always must be to better understand the students' strengths and weaknesses in their academic functioning in math, literacy, and other content-specific areas.

The four cases within this chapter are designed to highlight various ways in which school psychologists can engage in the support of children's academic development. The cases highlight a range of different academic difficulties and include a wide range of age/grade levels to allow discussions regard-ing appropriate types of responses to many different types of situations. The first case focuses on the support that a school psychologist provided a child through effective intervention design after utilizing CBM data to fully under-stand the area of concern within mathematics. The second case involves a student with a writing difficulty and focuses on how school psychologists can intervene to support academic progress in writing. The final two cases both focus on reading, with the third case focusing on a younger child and the fourth case focusing on an older child with reading-related concerns impact-ing academic progress.

Case One: Math Skill by Treatment Interaction

The school psychologist intern, Ms. Jenkins, was listening in a grade-level team problem-solving meeting as the team was discussing their concern for a student, Jordan, who scored low on the recent math benchmark assessments.

Jordan has lived in the United States since he was 2 years old when his family immigrated from Vietnam. Jordan speaks only English, although he reportedly understands his parents when they communicate with him in Vietnamese at home.

His teachers report that he is consistently failing his class unit tests and scored below the 10th percentile overall (see Table 3.1). Jordan's conceptual understanding scores on the benchmark were in the 31st percentile, slightly below average. Jordan's computation skills were in the 11th percentile range, well below average. At the end of the meeting, the intern offered her support to help provide a math intervention for Jordan. The teachers were thrilled to have extra help for the student.

Ms. Jenkins asked the teachers if she could review his recent assessments and classwork to assess his specific skills and needs. Upon reviewing his classwork, she noticed that he consistently made errors in addition with regrouping. After inspecting the data, Ms. Jenkins felt that the Concept-Representational-Abstract (CRA, EBI Network, 2014) intervention that she had learned about in her recent class might be an appropriate intervention to try with Jordan. She had read about the importance of the instructional hierarchy and skill by treatment interaction (Burns et al., 2010) in her earlier coursework and thought this might be a good opportunity to try to apply those theories in her own problem-solving. Based on the instructional hierarchy, CRA is an acquisition level intervention, which she felt would strengthen his conceptual understanding first. She collected more specific baseline with the student first by administering double-digit addition with regrouping CBM probes. In a two-minute probe, the student scored about two-digits correct per minute with 50 percent accuracy. She proceeded to meet with the student individually three times per week for 20-minutes per session. In that time, she

Table 3.1 Student Math Benchmark Assessment Fall to Spring

Third Grade	Fall Benchmark: Form A		Spring Benchmark: Form B	
	Standard Score	Percentile Rank	Standard Score	Percentile Rank
Concepts	90	31	80	10
Computation	81	11	87	18
Application	75	6	85	14
Total	80	9	88	17

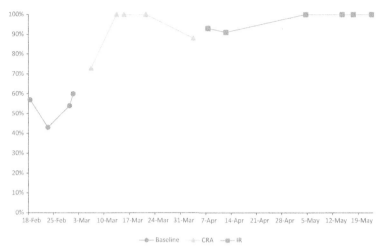

Figure 3.1 Percent Accuracy on Double Digit Addition With Regrouping

wrote a problem on a white board and provided base-ten blocks for the student to visually represent the equation. After Jordan completed the problem correctly, Ms. Jenkins would give Jordan five more similar problems to complete with feedback. The base-ten blocks were used to represent the problem and corrective feedback was provided. Jordan made immediate improvement with this strategy. Accuracy improved to 100 percent (see Figure 3.1). Fluency also improved but was still not at grade-level.

Based on the data and her understanding of the instructional hierarchy, Ms. Jenkins decided to switch gears with the intervention. Once Jordan demonstrated strong conceptual understanding and accuracy, she felt it was time to switch to a fluency strategy. Ms. Jordan then moved to the Incremental Rehearsal strategy (IR, Evidence Based Intervention Network, 2014; Burns, 2005) for fluency/proficiency, math flashcard practice with a ratio of 90 percent known problems and 10 percent unknown repeatedly interspersed. After switching to the IR strategy, the student made steady progress on the computation fluency goal (see Figure 3.2).

At the next benchmark assessment in the spring, Jordan had made progress overall, moving from a total score in the 9th percentile to the 17th percentile (see Table 3.1). Despite the rapid progress on fluency and accuracy of computation, the student's computation benchmark increased from the 11th percentile to the 18th percentile, but not substantially. The student was still scoring below average. The teachers were thrilled with the progress and wanted to

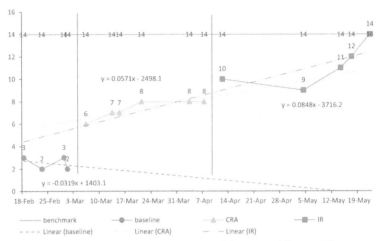

Figure 3.2 Correct Digits per Minute on Double Digit Addition With Regrouping

learn more about the strategies that were used. However, they were also still concerned about the student's benchmark assessments and unsure what to do next considering he was still so far behind on the spring benchmark. Ms. Jenkins realizes that she should seek out additional supervision from both her university-based and site-based supervisors to get additional ideas for how to continue supporting the teachers.

Discussion Questions

1. How did the use of assessment inform intervention decisions for this case? What types of assessment data were the most helpful for making intervention decisions? (**D1, D3**)
2. How might the team view the student differently if they only had the benchmark data, fall and spring, to review at their meetings and not the weekly progress monitoring data? (**D1**)
3. In this case, the intern provided direct service for the interventions. What are the advantages and disadvantages of direct academic service provision versus indirect? (**D2, D3**)
4. At the conclusion of the case, the teachers are excited about the intervention strategy. How should the intern proceed if she wants to begin

moving this case from direct services to indirect services to help give away the skills of the intervention and assessment? **(D2, D3)**

5. Given the data at the end of the case and teacher concerns, what should be the next steps? Is a special education evaluation warranted here? Why or why not? **(D1, D2, D3, D10)**
6. Are there cultural and language considerations that should be taken into consideration in this case? If yes, what should the team and Ms. Jenkins consider? **(D7)**
7. Ms. Jenkins is an intern so she continues to have access to supervision from both her university-based and site-based supervisors. However, once she completes her internship, she will likely not have access to the same types of mentorships. Why is it important to seek out mentors as a new school psychologist? What are suggestions for how to seek out support for professional development, consultation, and coaching in the role of the school psychologist? **(O3, O5, O6)**

Advanced Applications

1. Role play a conversation between the school psychology intern and the math teacher, reviewing the data graph, to determine the next steps. **(D1, D2, D3)**
2. Plan the next step for assessment. What curriculum-based measurement probes would you utilize next? Explain your rationale. **(D2)**
3. Role play a multidisciplinary meeting to review the progress-monitoring data and benchmark data to determine if further evaluation for special education services is needed. If yes, discuss what disability is suspected and what assessments or data would be needed given the referral concern. **(D1, D10)**

Case Two: Preempting Pre-Referral?

Mrs. Key, a long-time third-grade teacher, believed her student Amelia had a writing disability. Amelia is a third-grade student in Mrs. Key's class who identifies as White. Mrs. Key did not want to delay services to Amelia by following the school's pre-referral process, so she tried to work-around the school's typical process by sharing her concerns with Amelia's mother during her parent-teacher conference. Mrs. Key advised Amelia's mother to write a request for a meeting to discuss possible formal evaluation by the

Child Study Team. At the multidisciplinary team meeting, Ms. Dewmore, the school psychologist, recognized that no pre-referral problem-solving had been conducted prior to the meeting. She was concerned that without pre-referral problem-solving, including a trial of evidence-based interventions and progress monitoring data, the team would have a hard time ruling out lack of appropriate instruction as part of a determination of a specific learning disability in the area of writing. Ms. Dewmore did not feel comfortable proceeding to a formal evaluation without attempting this first. She offered to assist by conducting informal writing curriculum-based assessments (CBA) and curriculum-based measurements (CBM) to design and implement an intervention concurrent with an informal occupational-therapist (OT) and physical therapist (PT) screening for fine motor concerns. The team agreed and decided to reconvene in 6 weeks to allow time for an intervention trial period, with weekly data collection.

Ms. Dewmore consulted with Mrs. Key after the meeting. Reluctantly, Ms. Key agreed to meet weekly with Ms. Dewmore to work together via the Instructional Consultation (Rosenfield, 1987, 2014) process for Amelia's case. They met weekly and Ms. Key shared her concerns in more detail while also multitasking, including filing papers and grading. Ms. Dewmore tried to clarify and understand more about Amelia's skills. Ms. Key explained that Amelia's writing was illegible. Additionally, she was concerned about Amelia's reading comprehension and math fact fluency. Ms. Dewmore then conducted Instructional Assessments (Gickling et al., 2016) in reading, writing, and math to better analyze Amelia's skills and instructional starting points. Contrary to Mrs. Key's perspective, Amelia demonstrated strengths in both reading comprehension and math fact fluency. In reading comprehension, Amelia was able to verbally retell a grade-level reading passage in detail, she could also answer specific questions accurately about the text. Ms. Dewmore could see that legibility of her written responses to reading comprehension questions was likely what was making it difficult for Mrs. Key to accurately assess Amelia's comprehension skills. Amelia's written responses were illegible. In terms of the math fact fluency, it appeared that Amelia performed poorly on math computation assessments in class because the teacher was scoring illegible answers (e.g., number five written backwards) as incorrect even when the answer was technically accurate. Amelia's math fact computation was fast and accurate; however, the numbers were sometimes just transposed. It appeared that her handwriting was affecting her teacher's perception of her math accuracy.

After Ms. Dewmore shared the assessment results with Mrs. Key, they prioritized handwriting legibility, specifically correct letter and number formation, for intervention. Ms. Dewmore helped Ms. Key by collecting writing CBM data as a baseline and monitoring progress weekly. Mrs. Key did not have any new ideas as to what interventions would help. She said that she didn't teach handwriting until the end of third grade when they started the cursive unit. She also explained that they don't spend as much time on handwriting during the school day like they once did when she was a younger teacher. Ms. Dewmore conducted some research on handwriting development and interventions. She learned about a specific handwriting intervention (Graham et al., 2000) and shared that information with Mrs. Key. The intervention consisted of 15 minutes of handwriting instruction and fluency practice per day with letters that have similar formation strokes. This intervention did not address number formation, so Ms. Dewmore thought it would help to use prompt-fading worksheets for practicing the number five. She created worksheets where the number five had an outline of a cobra snake around the five to illustrate how you start at the head and trace around the body. The cobra outline was faded to tracing the five, then gradually to dotted lines and then freewriting the five.

Mrs. Key did not see any possible way that she could spend 15 minutes on this type of instruction given her busy class schedule. Ms. Dewmore was frustrated with Mrs. Key's resistance because she was concerned about Amelia's progress and wanted to have data to assess response to intervention. Ms. Dewmore pushed forward, despite some of these barriers and resistance from the teacher. She suggested that the intervention could be implemented by the paraeducator, not the classroom teacher. Mrs. Key agreed because it did not interfere in her own instruction and she could see how a few other students in her class could benefit from a similar intervention. They decided to create a small group for the paraeducator to work with to implement the handwriting intervention. The teacher did agree to use the math number five practice worksheets with Amelia as a warm-up in math class. She felt that this was easy to implement without significantly changing instructional time.

With these interventions in place, Amelia made rapid progress. Mrs. Key was pleasantly surprised by the noticeable changes to Amelia's writing in class. In fact, now that the teacher could read Amelia's writing, she thought Amelia may be advanced in writing, due to her creativity and expression. Mrs. Dewmore shared the graphed data and pre-post writing samples at the follow-up multidisciplinary team meeting (see Figure 3.3). The team decided no further formal evaluation was needed because the parent and teacher no longer suspected a disability. After the team meeting, Mrs. Key reflected about the value of the consultation process. She felt much more positive about pre-referral problem-solving as a result of her experience working with Ms. Dewmore.

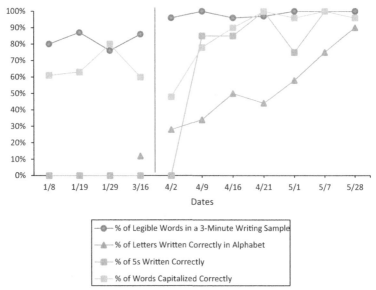

Figure 3.3 Percent of Legible Words in a 3-Minute Writing Sample

Discussion Questions

1. What might have happened if the school psychologist did not offer a collaborative consultation approach for this case? How might the outcomes for this student be different? (**D2**)

2. What could the consultant have done differently from an indirect service delivery perspective? What could be done in a future case with this teacher to emphasize the teacher outcomes of the case? (**D2, O1**)

3. Teachers judge students' writing content more negatively if there are significant legibility concerns (Graham et al., 2000) and handwriting is often not taught explicitly in schools as it once was. What is the school psychologist's role in sharing handwriting development and intervention information with teachers, providing professional development, and assisting with this type of intervention via consultation or coaching? (**D2, D3, D5**)

4. The parent seemed to be easily persuaded to view this as a special education or disability concern from the parent-teacher conference but was also equally open to trying other options first once presented by Ms. Dewmore. What does this mean for the role of school psychologist in

educating parents about the value of problem-solving prior to suspecting a disability, as well as what that process could look like? What would you suggest Ms. Dewmore do to educate parents in the school about pre-referral problem-solving? (**D2, D7, D10**)

Advanced Applications

1. Review the Graham et al. (2000) research article and create an intervention script for a teacher based on the description of the intervention in the article. (**D3, D9**)
2. Using that same intervention, create a method to assess intervention fidelity (e.g., an observation checklist, a teacher self-assessment checklist, permanent product review). (**D1, D2, D3, D9**)
3. Role-play a consultation conversation between Ms. Dewmore and Mrs. Key. In the role of Ms. Dewmore, plan to address the teacher multitasking in an open, but non-confrontational way, and to try to shift from more direct service to indirect service. What communication skills or motivational interviewing skills would be helpful here? (**D2**)
4. It would be helpful to be able to evaluate how consultative and indirect service delivery models impact student outcomes. How might the service delivery in this school be evaluated? (**O1**)

Case Three: Pitfalls and Plateaus

A school psychology intern, Ms. Eager, attended her first Student Support Team (SST) meeting at her internship site. At the meeting, she listened carefully to the referring teacher's concerns about her student, an English learner (EL), Mario. The teacher, Ms. Stewart, relayed her concerns to the team about his lack of reading progress and work completion. She said, "He just won't do the work! I think he's going to need more intensive services." Trying to better understand the concerns, Ms. Eager asked the referring teacher a clarifying question. Ms. Eager asks, "What is the work that Mario is having trouble completing?" Another teacher on the team rushed to Ms. Stewart's defense saying, "Oh no! She knows her students!" She appeared offended that Ms. Eager would question the teacher. Ms. Eager recognized that she must have overstepped as a newcomer to the school. She apologized and explained that she wasn't questioning the teacher's judgment and was just trying to get a clearer picture of the concern.

After the meeting, Ms. Eager went to Ms. Stewart to check-in and apologize again. She also offered consultative services. The teacher agreed to meet weekly prior to the next scheduled SST follow-up meeting. After collecting some data on Mario's reading skills and needs, they prioritized letter and sound identification, focusing on folding-in one letter and sound at a time with a high number of repetitions daily. Mario started making progress, with an immediate increase in letter recognition on the graph that Ms. Eager was helping the teacher to create weekly (see Figure 3.4).

Weeks later, Mario missed a few weeks of school due to a broken leg. Then, Ms. Stewart missed a few weeks of school due to an elective surgery. When she returned, Ms. Stewart was concerned about Mario's lack of progress (see Figure 3.4). She felt he had plateaued for several weeks. Ms. Stewart wanted to refer Mario for a special education evaluation. Ms. Eager agreed that the data indicated a plateau. However, she recognized that this plateau may be due to lack of consistent implementation of the intervention, while the teacher and student were both absent at different times, Ms. Eager showed Ms. Stewart a graph with vertical lines indicating implementation stops and starts to help the teacher connect the lack of progress with lack of implementation. Ms. Eager shared information with Ms. Stewart about the exclusionary criteria for specific-learning disability, including lack of appropriate instruction, as well as the long-term process of language acquisition for EL students, including the differences between the acquisition of interpersonal communication skills and cognitive and academic language proficiency.

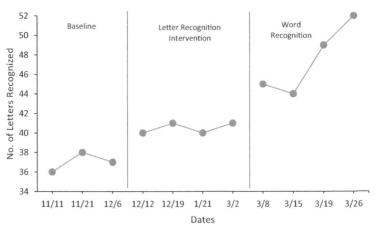

Figure 3.4 Case Progress Data: Number of Upper and Lowercase Letters Recognized

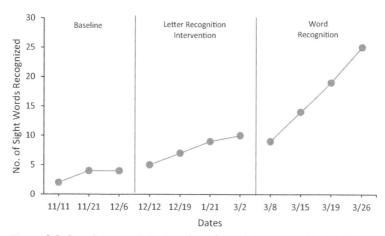

Figure 3.5 Case Progress Data: Number of Words Recognized by Sight

Ms. Stewart agreed that they should focus on implementation before returning to the team, to rule out lack of intervention. Ms. Stewart was concerned about the lack of reading progress and the amount of time that had passed, so they also switched the intervention design to a word-level intervention, in hopes of boosting his progress. They now used the folding-in technique for word recognition, rather than letter/sound recognition, via "pocket cards," and reading words in context of a "teacher-made story" with the target words and known words (Gickling et al., 2016). The student made rapid progress with words and letter/sounds once they switched to this intervention, even with stopping the letter/sound intervention (see Figures 3.4 and 3.5). It appeared that the student was making more sense of letters and sounds once they were learned within the context of learning words. The teacher began to realize that this student could learn quickly with the right intervention and implementation. They shared progress with the team and decided no further evaluation or services would be needed.

Discussion Questions

1.   Although Ms. Eager asked an innocuous question, what went wrong in her first interaction? **(D2)**
2.   How did Ms. Eager have to repair potential relationship damage from the initial perceived misstep at the meeting? **(D2)**

3. What did the teacher's reactions at the team meeting indicate about the culture of the school regarding beliefs around student problems and/or how academic problems are solved? What about the teacher's quickness to refer for special education evaluation after lack of progress? What can be done about that as a school psychologist? (**D2, D5, O2**)
4. Why was it critical that Ms. Eager visually displayed intervention phase lines on the graph to indicate when the intervention stopped and started? (**D1**)
5. Discuss the cultural aspects of this case. Why was it important that Ms. Eager introduce a problem-solving approach for this case in particular? Why might it have been more effective to switch to working on words rather than letters/sounds for this student? (**D8, D3**)
6. Discuss the legal aspects of this case. What are the inclusionary and exclusionary criteria of specific learning disability? (**D10**)

Advanced Applications

1. Create an intervention script and treatment fidelity measure for the folding-in or "drill sandwich" intervention (Gickling et al., 2016). (**D1, D3**)
2. Role play the conversation with the teacher around the data plateau, her concerns, and next steps. (**D2**)
3. Plan a faculty in-service session introducing your role as a school consultant, supporting academic interventions and instructional support. Include rationale for the importance of a problem-solving approach prior to or during the special education referral process (**D5, D10, O1, O4, O5**)
4. Within the case, there is a mention of the long-term process associated with acquiring a second language with proficiency in cognitive and academic language. Research the process of second language acquisition. With knowledge of that long-term process, analyze how schools should consider second language acquisition for EL children who are considered by the school to be behind academically. (**D1, D8**)

Case Four: "Dystaughtia"

Kenya's mother, Ms. Chapman, is increasingly becoming concerned now that Kenya is in high school and is still significantly struggling in reading. Kenya, a Black female, is starting her sophomore year in high school in a suburban school district, in a predominantly white school. Kenya has struggled with reading for several years now. It wasn't apparent to Ms. Chapman at first because Kenya had a strong start in Kindergarten and was on or above grade level at times, according to her teacher. Kenya loved her Kindergarten teacher. Her mother was also very pleased with that teacher because she could tell she was a highly effective teacher. The teacher was so effective that she left the Kindergarten team to become the Reading Specialist for the school. Kenya's reading difficulties did not start to appear until about second or third grade. Ms. Chapman was concerned that Kenya had inconsistent reading instruction during those years because throughout the time she had long-term substitute teachers due to teacher maternity leave or other reasons. At the time, Ms. Chapman couldn't believe the odds of having that happen three years in a row. She hoped it didn't matter, but always wondered if that was part of Kenya's difficulty with reading. By the time Kenya was in the fifth grade, her reading difficulties were very clear to Ms. Chapman. Kenya's reading benchmark scores were well below grade level in the fall of that year. In early fall, after seeing the score report, Ms. Chapman requested a Student Support Team (SST) meeting to raise her concerns.

At the SST meeting, the fifth-grade teachers all reported that Kenya was a positive, cooperative, and a sweet child. They did not appear overly concerned about her reading level. The teachers felt that she could do better academically if she would just focus more. They felt she was task-avoidant at times and thought that was getting in the way of her reading achievement. They mentioned that she would talk to her peers and would need to be redirected frequently to do her work. After hearing Ms. Chapman's concern about reading, they agreed to offer Kenya some reading support. The SST plan indicated that she would get reading intervention. The intervention plan was for Kenya to come in during lunch to read with a peer during lunch and play sight-word games one time per week. They also said that a paraprofessional would work with Kenya one additional time per week on reading strategies. Kenya's mother was skeptical that this would help and was not quite sure what to say or how to advocate for something more or different. She did not want to "rock the boat," so felt it would be best to give the team a little time to try their suggestions.

At the follow-up SST meeting, in the winter, the teachers reported that Kenya was doing well. They felt she was making good progress because she was getting 80–90 percent on the reading assignments in class. Ms. Chapman was concerned because according to the winter benchmark assessment report that was sent home, Kenya's scores appeared to be about the same as the fall. Ms. Chapman was hoping there would be other weekly progress monitoring data to review other than teacher input or quiz grades. It did not make sense to her that Kenya could perform well on quizzes, but then perform so poorly on benchmark assessments. She felt that it must be a sign of other reading difficulties. Kenya's mother had read online about the Response to Intervention (RTI) approach. She asked if the school had been graphing data weekly to monitor progress. The school psychologist said, "oh we do RTI, we just don't do the data graphing part." Ms. Chapman felt frustrated and a bit helpless about what to do to advocate with the school team for what she thought might be better. She was not convinced at all that the agreed-upon intervention plan had even been implemented. However, the team felt it was important to stay the course. At the next SST meeting, the spring benchmark data were available and Kenya's score declined slightly from winter to spring. In fact, she was now scoring below the 10th percentile in the reading assessment. At that point, her mother was adamant that something different must be done.

After agreeing to a special education evaluation, at the beginning of sixth grade, Kenya was found eligible for special education as a student with a Specific Learning Disability in Reading. The school psychologist shared the data from her report. See Tables 3.2, 3.3, and 3.4.

The school psychologist's report stated that Kenya was a student who had average cognitive abilities with significant deficits in working memory and

Table 3.2 Summary of WISC-V Composite/Index Scores

Scale	Index/ Composite Standard Score	Percentile Rank	95% Confidence Interval	Qualitative Description
Verbal Comprehension Index (VCI)	93	30	85–100	Average
Visual-Spatial Index (VSI)	83	14	78–93	Low Average
Fluid Reasoning Index (FRI)	101	50	93–107	Average
Working Memory Index (WMI)	81	12	76–92	Low Average
Processing Speed Index (PSI)	110	77	101–119	High Average
Full Scale IQ	93	32	88–99	Average

Table 3.3 Bender Gestalt-II Summary: Visual Motor Integration Skills

	Copy	Recall
Standard Score	94	114
Percentile Rank	34	82
Description	Average	High Average

Table 3.4 Woodcock Johnson IV: Academic Achievement Assessment

Standard Battery	Standard Scores	Grade Equivalent
Letter Word Identification	87	4.0
Applied Problems	75	3.1
Spelling	93	5.1
Passage Comprehension	80	3.1
Calculation	86	4.4
Writing Samples	100	6.9
Word Attack	86	3.1
Sentence Reading Fluency	86	4.0
Math Facts Fluency	102	6.6
Sentence Writing Fluency	92	5.0
CLUSTERS	Standard Scores	Grade Equivalent
Reading	83	
Broad Reading	83	
Basic Reading Skills	85	
Mathematics	81	
Written Language	96	

visual spatial skills as compared with processing speed. In terms of academic skills, Kenya was found to be in the low average to average range. The school psychologist indicated that Kenya's deficits in working memory and spatial abilities could have a significant impact on her ability to learn and may explain her low average achievement in reading and math.

In that first year of middle school, and with the newly developed IEP, Kenya's teachers continued to report that she was positive, social, and "a pleasure to have in class." Kenya did well in most of her classes except those with a heavy reading and writing load. In the first quarter of sixth grade, she had a D in Science and Social Studies, and was failing Language Arts. Kenya received special education reading intervention services in a reading intervention class period, in lieu of an arts elective. During that class, she received computer-assisted reading intervention. Her mother was concerned because, once again, Kenya's reading teacher was out for a long-term leave. This time it was a medical leave. Her mother did not want to complain because she felt genuine concern for the teacher on leave, but at the same time she was worried. The new reading intervention teacher was a long-term substitute teacher who was not specifically trained in reading. At the end of the sixth-grade year, Kenya was doing well in terms of grades, but her spring benchmark score remained at around the 10th percentile. Seventh-grade was similar for Kenya. The same reading intervention teacher continued to have medical concerns and Kenya's substitute continued to rely on computer-assisted intervention during that class period. At the annual review IEP meeting, Kenya's teachers praised her for being a hard-working student and earning good grades. Kenya's mother was pleased to hear how well her daughter was adjusting to middle school and that she continued to do well socially and in terms of her grades, yet she was increasingly frustrated about the continued lack of actual reading progress on formal district benchmark assessments.

At the annual IEP review, at the end of Kenya's seventh-grade year, Ms. Chapman asks the team for more specific assessment data to try to understand why Kenya continues to do well in class, but not on major assessments. The team did not feel more assessment would yield new or different results. Knowing something was not working for Kenya, Ms. Chapman tried shifting to changing the IEP services to be more specific. She noticed that the IEP goals felt very vague and perhaps were not targeting the areas that Kenya needed the most help. One goal said,

> After reading a short story with a partner or group of peers, Kenya will complete an interactive notebook entry with 2 pieces of text evidence and verbally describe the main characters using 2 pieces of text evidence, one explicit and one implicit to support her analysis in 4 out of 5 trials with 80% accuracy.

Ms. Chapman was most worried about the report that indicated her daughter was reading at a third-grade level in terms of word attack. There were no goals for word-attack skills. There was also no special instruction on the IEP for anything related to phonics. Ms. Chapman tried asking for that to be written into the IEP. The school psychologist replied, "It is not our job as a team to dictate instruction." Ms. Chapman was speechless and unsure how to push for more at that moment. She thought that was the legal purpose of the team, but was not sure how to ask for more without sounding adversarial. Even if she spoke up, she felt the team was not understanding what she was asking for or did not know what else to do. She was at a loss.

Luckily, the school district started a new program during Kenya's eighth-grade year. They implemented a universal screening tool, the Advanced Decoding Survey (Really Great Reading©, 2013). Special educators from the school district administered the screening and informed the school of the students who qualified for a phonics intervention. Kenya qualified for services based on her scores. From the survey, Kenya scored in the "low" range for multisyllabic decoding skills and "emerging" for advanced vowel sounds. The district trained the special educators in an explicit phonics manualized intervention program. Kenya would now receive this phonics program during her reading intervention program time, by the special educator trained in this program, rather than the computer-program with the long-term substitute teacher during reading intervention time. To no surprise to Ms. Chapman, Kenya was finally making progress in reading. There was a small bump up at the end of the year benchmark after many years of no progress.

Kenya transitioned to high school the next year and made the social transition well. Once again, her teachers all felt she was a pleasure to have in class and was a hard-worker. She was on honor roll for the first two quarters of the school year, so they had no concerns. Ms. Chapman was thrilled with her daughter's ability to manage the challenge of high school, especially given how hard she knew her daughter had to work to achieve that level of success. At the same time, Ms. Chapman was anxious about her daughter's future because on her recent PSAT score report, her daughter scored in the 4th percentile. Ms. Chapman knows that without strong reading skills her daughter will have a very difficult time getting into college and staying afloat once she is in college. Kenya said that her guidance counselor has been talking to her about non-college career paths. Ms. Chapman wants her daughter to know she can take any path that she wants, but she does not want to close the door on college options. Ms. Chapman knows how quickly her daughter can learn, if she has the right instruction.

At the Annual IEP review meeting, at the end of the ninth-grade year, Ms. Chapman was alarmed to hear that Kenya had not been receiving any reading intervention services. She had not realized that this was not a part of her schedule or program. Ms. Chapman just assumed that it would continue at the new school. The school team were very quick to make the situation right and arranged for immediate reading intervention services for Kenya, but almost a year had passed with no services. The team readministered the Advanced Decoding Survey and Kenya scored very similar to the year prior. Ms. Chapman was upset to have lost so much time and felt like they were starting again from square one. She realized the explicit phonics program that had been added in eighth grade was never written directly into the IEP so it must have been missed in the transition to high school. She requested that specific phonics goals be added to the IEP and phonics intervention for the advanced vowels and multisyllabic word decoding. The team was reluctant to provide any specific program name in the IEP, but did agree to add a goal, "Given a list of 30 multisyllabic words, Kenya will read the words with automaticity and with 80% accuracy." Ms. Chapman was glad to see that they added the decoding goal, so felt that was a step in the right direction. She left the meeting thinking there may still be something not quite right with an 80 percent goal, but she was not sure what to say about that to the team. In her mind, Kenya would need to be able to read with a much higher accuracy level to truly comprehend what she is reading in class and in real life, but she second-guessed herself at the meeting and did not know how much further she could push back being newer to this high school team.

Discussion Questions

1. What assessment issues are present in this case? What are concerns about some of the specific assessment measures used in this evaluation? (**D1**)
2. What legal issues are present in this case? (**D10**)
3. Was the school psychologist correct in saying it is not the team's job to dictate instruction? Why or why not? (**D3, D10, O4**)
4. What is the role of the IEP Team in regards to determining specialized instruction? (**D3, D10**)
5. What intervention issues are present in this case? (**D3**)
6. Kenya was receiving reading intervention services in a separate class from Language Arts. She was failing Language Arts. What other supports might have been needed in addition to a reading intervention class? What is the school psychologist's role in connecting those dots? (**D2, D3, D10**)
7. What is the school psychologist's role in consulting with the teachers before and after the meeting in this case? If you were the school

psychologist, how would you have followed-up with the teachers or staff after each meeting? (**D2**)

8. How did communication in the meetings or after the meetings affect parent/school relationships? How might listening to the parent have improved student outcomes? (**D2, D7**)

9. In almost every meeting throughout the years, Ms. Chapman feels unsure and/or unheard. She consistently tries to advocate for her daughter, yet she hits many roadblocks from school-based team members. In what specific ways did the team members contribute to these roadblocks? What specifically could have been done differently in these meetings? (**D7**)

10. Discuss the cultural considerations in this case. How might racial bias of the team members have played a role here? What actions may have contributed to disproportionate special education placement for students of color at this school? What could have been done to prevent a potentially unnecessary special education placement? (**D8**)

Advanced Applications

1. If you were the school psychologist for this case, what assessment steps would you have taken? What specific assessments would you recommend? Why? (**D1**)

2. Read information on the use of age versus grade equivalencies (e.g., Reynolds, 1981; Smith, 2009). Which should the school psychologist have reported and why? (**D1**)

3. Evaluate how the data was presented in the report tables. What recommendations would you make for revisions to the data report format? (**D1**)

4. Review the research on computer-assisted interventions for reading. What programs are evidence-based and meet the needs presented in this case, if any? (**D3, D9**)

5. Review the research on phonics intervention, specifically for the phonics skills indicated as a need in the later assessment in this case. What interventions or programs are evidence-based and meet the needs presented in this case? (**D3, D9**)

6. Discuss and determine what a more effective IEP goal would be for this case, for the phonics concern. What are the limitations of the current goal? Write a new goal that addresses those concerns. What measure would you recommend for progress monitoring? What frequency would you suggest this data to be collected? Explain your rationale. (**D1**)

7. Review the eligibility criteria for a Specific Learning Disability in your state. Would you have qualified this student for special education services, given this information? If no, why not? If yes, using which model, the discrepancy model, response to intervention, or patterns of strengths and weaknesses? Did the student meet the inclusionary criteria? Did the student meet the exclusionary criteria? How would you determine if cultural, environmental, or lack of appropriate instruction? (**D1, D10**)

8. Scholars have written about the over-identification of Black students in the category of Specific Learning Disability, as well as the potential underrepresentation of research on Black students in reading intervention research (Proctor et al., 2012; Robinson, 2013). Review the research on this and discuss if or how it might relate to this case. What are the implications for school psychologists? (**D3, D8**)

References

Burns, M. K. (2005). Using incremental rehearsal to increase fluency of single digit multiplication facts with children identified as learning disabled in mathematics computation. *Education and Treatment of Children, 28*(3), 237–249.

Burns, M. K., Codding, R. S., Boice, C. H., & Lukito, G. (2010). Meta-analysis of acquisition and fluency math interventions with instructional and frustrational level skills: Evidence for a skill-by-treatment interaction. *School Psychology Review, 39*(1), 69–83. www.jstor.org/stable/42899847

Evidence Based Intervention Network. (2014, January 30). *Concrete-representational-abstract (CRA).* Retrieved September 1, 2020, from https://ebi.missouri.edu/?p=1006

Gickling, E. E., Gravois, T. A., & Angels, V. (2016). *Instructional assessment: An essential path for Guiding reading instruction.* ICAT Publishing.

Graham, S., Harris, K. R., & Fink, B. (2000). Is handwriting causally related to learning to write? Treatment of handwriting problems in beginning writers. *Journal of Educational Psychology, 92*(4), 620–633. https://doi.org/10.1037/0022-0663.92.4.620

National Association of School Psychology. (2020). *The professional standards of the national association of school psychologists.* National Association of School Psychologists.

Proctor, S. L., Graves, S. L., & Esch, R. C. (2012). Assessing African American students for specific learning disabilities: The promises and perils of response to intervention. *The Journal of Negro Education, 81*(3), 268–282. https://doi.org/10.7709/jnegroeducation.81.3.0268

Really Great Reading©. (2013). *Advanced decoding survey plus.* www.reallygreatreading.com/rgrdownloads/really_great_reading_ads_plus.pdf

Reynolds, C. R. (1981). The fallacy of "two years below grade level for age" as a criterion for reading disorders. *The Journal of School Psychology, 19*(4), 350–358. https://doi.org/10.1016/0022-4405(81)90029-7

Robinson, S. A. (2013). Educating Black males with dyslexia. *Interdisciplinary Journal of Teaching and Learning, 3*(3), 159–174.

Rosenfield, S. A. (1987). *Instructional consultation*. Lawrence Erlbaum Associates.

Rosenfield, S. A. (2014). Best practices in instructional consultation and instructional consultation teams. In P. L. Harrison & A. Thomas (Eds.), *Best practices in school psychology: Data-based and collaborative decision making* (pp. 509–524). National Association of School Psychologists.

Smith, M. (2009). *The Hippocratic Oath and grade equivalents*. http://cdn.lexile.com/m/uploads/positionpapers/TheHippOathandGrdEquiv.pdf

Providing Services in Mental and Behavioral Health Services

4

Domain 4: Mental and Behavioral Health Services

"School psychologists understand the biological, cultural, developmental, and social influences on mental and behavioral health, behavioral and emotional impacts on learning, and evidence-based strategies to promote social—emotional functioning. School psychologists, in collaboration with others, design, implement, and evaluate services that promote resilience and positive behavior, support socialization and adaptive skills, and enhance mental and behavioral health." (NASP, 2020, p. 5)

School psychologists operate as mental health professionals in schools. They utilize their knowledge and skills in mental health, child development, and behavioral development to advocate within schools for evidence-based interventions to support the social, emotional, and behavioral development of all children. This involves understanding the connection between behavioral and mental health on academic functioning, utilizing developmentally appropriate assessment and intervention strategies with children, and advocating for evidence-based, school-wide programming to support the social, emotional, behavioral, and mental health of all children. The four cases in this chapter focus on various ways in which school psychologists might be involved in mental and behavioral health services for children.

Examples of how school psychologists can support all children along a continuum of supports are provided by NASP (2020) and include various types of school-based counseling. This may involve individual counseling, group counseling, and various types of skill development (i.e., social skills groups). A focus on the development of effective social and emotional skills, such as "self-regulation, self-monitoring, self-advocacy, planning/organization, empathy, positive coping strategies, interpersonal skills, and healthy decision making" (NASP, 2020, pp. 5–6) is imperative in schools. School psychologists have key knowledge and skills to assist in the development of these skills. The first two cases in this chapter illustrate the need for these different types of counseling services to meet a variety of student needs. Cases One and Two focus on externalizing concerns such as physical and verbal aggression. Case two, "Mounting Pressures," takes a closer look at how externalizing problems may be masking internalizing issues like anxiety. These cases allow for reflection and analysis of the various counseling theories and techniques that might be appropriate for use in school-based counseling sessions. Case Four, "When the Pandemic Comes Along," also allows for discussion of the long-term impact of the pandemic on students' mental health (as well as academic progress) and what services may be needed.

School psychologists also must utilize appropriate assessment techniques to guide problem-solving, not only to identify students in need of support, but also to understand child functioning, including through the adoption of an ecological perspective of the impact of environmental factors, such as trauma, on children's development. In Case One, "Screening for Intervention," a universal screening measure of verbal and aggressive behaviors is implemented across a grade-level to identify and provide targeted support to students who were found to be at-risk for aggression. In Case Four, grades are used as a data-point to indicate a change in student performance and need for further intervention. Case Three, "Class-wide Intervention," utilizes behavioral observation data, at the classroom level, to identify ecological factors to target for classroom-systems-level intervention. The same data was then used to monitor implementation fidelity and progress. School psychologists are also critical to ensuring effective implementation of interventions. Cases one and three allow for the discussion of how to assess and support both treatment acceptability and treatment integrity of interventions that are implemented within the school setting.

School psychologists might be involved in the implementation of class-wide and/or school-wide social-emotional learning programs, parent education, parent support, and class and school-wide positive behavioral support. Cases One and Three illustrate those types of systems-level direct and indirect mental and behavioral health interventions. To work within a systems-level orientation, school psychologists must also be effective in collaborating with various community agencies, mental health professionals and other medical professionals in providing comprehensive services for children in need of robust social, emotional, and behavioral supports. Similarly, school psychologists should seek to develop positive relationships with families to ensure effective collaboration and coordination of services for children, while also striving to strengthen the home-school connection. Cases One, Two, and Four provide opportunities to analyze home-school collaboration, while Case Three focuses more specifically on teacher consultation.

Each case provides opportunities to reflect on the cultural, developmental, and social influences on academic performance in school. Cases One and Two explicitly allow for open discussion around cultural dynamics, such as potential implicit biases or stereotypes. All the cases span different developmental levels from middle childhood (Case Three), early adolescence (Cases One and Four), to late adolescence (Case Two). Case Four provides a unique opportunity to discuss current social influences affecting development, namely the health pandemic and abrupt shift to virtual instruction, which may influence academic and social functioning.

Case One: Screening for Intervention

A large, urban middle school in a major United States city was interested in reducing aggressive behaviors of their students and helping students cope with anger in more positive and prosocial ways. To this end, the school decided to collect screening data at the end of the sixth-grade year to determine needs for a large-scale, seventh grade social-emotional learning intervention. This middle school was diverse in that 45 percent of students identified as Black, 30 percent of students identified as Hispanic, 20 percent of students identified as White, with the remaining 5 percent identifying as Other. The school had a large proportion of students (70 percent) who qualified for Free and Reduced Meals (FARMS). The school historically has had concerns with the behavior of many students. Punitive discipline measures are routine in the school, with a large percentage of students (65 percent) having been suspended with either in-school or out-of-school suspension in the past two years. The administrators have reported that many of the disciplinary actions are related to physical aggression, verbal aggression (towards peers and/or teachers), disrespect to teachers, and noncompliance with teacher rules.

The screening measure focused on physical and verbal aggression towards peers and adults and included a 15-item teacher survey that included a five-point Likert scale format (1=Strongly Disagree, 2=Disagree, 3=Neutral, 4=Agree, 5=Strongly Agree). A letter was sent home to parents indicating that this survey would be distributed at the end of the year to all sixth-grade students, unless the parents signed the form and returned it to the school indicating that they did not want their child's teacher to complete the survey for their child. The school only received five letters back from parents indicating that they did not want the survey completed about their child. The results of the screening indicated that 60 of the 200 students in sixth grade (30 percent of the grade) met the pre-determined cut-off score that indicated that they were at-risk for demonstrating physical and verbal aggression towards others. Of these 60 at-risk students, 70 percent were Black students, 23 percent were Hispanic students, and 7 percent were Caucasian students. Additionally, 97 percent of the students identified were males.

Over the summer, it was decided to group these 60 students who were determined to be at-risk into groups of 10 for small group anger management sessions for the seventh grade. The composition of each group of 10 was largely based on their academic schedules and students were grouped together based on their elective and study hall schedule to minimize disruption to any of the core academic classes.

The school psychologist and the school counselor researched and selected an anger management program to use. They hypothesized that the activities presented in this curriculum would be engaging to middle school students and felt that the materials would be easy to follow along with for them as group leaders. When the groups began in the fall for the identified seventh graders, the school psychologist and school counselor met regularly to discuss the progress of the groups. To their surprise some of the groups seemed to be going well with the students engaged and motivated to attend, while other groups had the complete opposite experience, and the children seemed disengaged and unmotivated. Some of the children in those groups indicated that they no longer wanted to attend the group. Several parents had already called the school asking why their children were in these groups and expressing that their children did not want to participate any longer. The school psychologist and school counselor could not understand why this group seemed to be working well in some of the groups, but not in other groups.

Discussion Questions

1. What are the ethical considerations for running this group? (**D10**)
2. What are some of the issues presented here regarding passive consent for the teacher ratings of aggressive behaviors? Is active consent from parents needed for students to be involved in the actual anger management groups? (**D10**)
3. What might be some iatrogenic effects of grouping students together? (**D10**)
4. Specifically, how might the few females have identified for participation in these groups fare as participants? What hypotheses do you have about their potential willingness to be part of these groups? (**D8**)
5. What process should the school psychologist and the school counselor have taken for identifying the best intervention for this group? (**D9**)
6. What cultural considerations are needed prior to selecting and implementing an intervention such as this one? (**D8**)
7. What might the screening data suggest about teacher perceptions about student aggression in the school? What alternate ecological hypotheses could be made about the aggressive behavior? How might changing the hypothesis, alter your decisions about interventions? (**D8**)
8. What should the school psychologist do to engage teachers in intervention efforts and to promote skill generalization? (**D2, O4**)
9. How should the school psychologist and school counselor connect with families to gain consent, engage, and promote skill generalization? (**D7**)
10. Review the research by Pas et al. (2020) about attendance patterns with Tier II and Tier III interventions. How might the school psychologist and school counselor use these findings to conceptualize the attendance problems that they are facing in their groups? (**D4, D9**)

Advanced Applications

1. The school's original idea to focus on reducing disciplinary issues related to verbal and physical aggression is a potentially positive one. Design a plan for how the school teams should go about assessing factors associated with the disciplinary problems in the school. What types of needs assessments or data collection might be necessary? (**D9**).
2. Research some anger management counseling programs that might be implemented with whole-classes, small groups or even a whole school approach. Identify some programs and provide information about the

pros and cons of each program (**D4**). Consider cultural implications for each. (**D8**).

3. What specific types of professional development for the teachers, administrators and mental health professionals in the school might be necessary to ensure effective service delivery of this new program? (**O6**)

4. Review the "Best Practices in Group Counseling" chapter by Herbstrith and Tobin (2014). Apply some of the practices suggested for use in this case.

Case Two: Mounting Pressures

Christopher is a male 11th-grade student of Korean descent who has been referred for counseling with the school psychologist, Ms. Randall, by both the assistant principal and Christopher's parents. According to his mother, Christopher has always excelled in school and has had no difficulties meeting expectations in various challenging classes. In fact, this year, Christopher is taking three advanced placement classes, and three honors classes so he can improve his chances of admission to an elite college. He also reportedly has never had any discipline issues in school. However, now it is November of his junior year of high school and there have been four disciplinary incidents. All the incidents are related to Christopher becoming overly emotional and angry during school. In two of these incidents, he angrily yelled at a teacher after receiving a B on an assignment that he believed was an unfair grade. As a result of these incidents, he was sent to the office with a discipline referral for class disruption and disrespect towards the teacher.

In another incident, Christopher was found crying uncontrollably in the library by the librarian. He refused to provide any information to the librarian about what was wrong and refused to move from the spot that he was in for approximately 45 minutes, which resulted in him receiving a discipline referral for skipping his next class. The latest incident occurred after Christopher met with his guidance counselor about the college application process. Christopher reportedly angrily kicked the counselor's desk and stormed out of the office, leaving school grounds for approximately 20 minutes before returning. The counselor indicated that she had been describing the application process for college to Christopher and asking him about potential majors when this outburst occurred, seemingly out of the blue. This incident was deemed by the assistant principal to be a more serious disciplinary issue because Christopher left school grounds, which is a safety concern. In fact, multiple school officials, including the school resource officer (SRO) were involved in searching for Christopher during this time period until he eventually returned to the school on his own. He indicated that he just needed to take a walk to calm down and that he didn't mean to break any school rules. Due to the seriousness of this incident, Christopher was suspended from school for two days. During his suspension, Ms. Randall called home and spoke with both Christopher and his mother. His mother reported that he was grounded at home because of the issues he had at school. She also reported that she was at a loss regarding why he would be behaving this way. The school psychologist asked if she could speak to Christopher and his mother indicated that she would attempt to get him on the phone. Somewhat surprisingly, Christopher willingly came to the phone and immediately began sharing some of his concerns. He indicated that he feels "like no one understands me" and reported feeling immense pressure and anxiety about his future plans. Christopher agreed to come to a counseling session with Ms. Randall and the first session will occur upon Christopher's return to school from his suspension.

Discussion Questions

1. What additional information might the school psychologist want to gather prior to her first counseling session with Christopher? (**D1**)
2. Provide some ideas of how the counseling session with Christopher can be started. What would be some goals for the first session? (**D4**)
3. What are some hypotheses that the school psychologist might have regarding the nature of Christopher's sudden behavioral problems? What might be the source of his behavioral issue at school? (**D4**)
4. Thus far, the focus of the school and his parents seem to be disciplinary and punitive in nature. How effective do you think the disciplinary actions taken by the school will be in improving Christopher's behavior? Why? (**D5**)
5. Christopher has already reported to the school psychologist that he doesn't feel that anybody understands him. How might this be used in the initial counseling sessions to further understand how Christopher is currently feeling? (**D4**)
6. By your sixth session with Christopher, he is comfortable expressing that he feels enormous pressure to get into an elite University. He reports that some of this pressure comes from the expectations of his parents since they are both successful in their chosen fields, but it mostly comes from the pressure that he is putting on himself. He reports to the school psychologist that he feels like he might be happier if he goes to community college after high school instead of applying to four-year colleges. He

specifically asks for advice and asks if he should take this route. How might the school psychologist respond? (**D4**)

7. What are potential cultural considerations or issues in this case? Should cultural variables be considered? Why or why not? (**D8**)

Advanced Applications

1. Select three counseling <u>theories</u> and explore how counseling sessions might proceed when using those theories in counseling Christopher. (**D4**)
2. Select three different specific counseling <u>techniques</u> that might be considered for use with Christopher at some point in the counseling relationship. (**D4**)
3. It might be helpful to also include consultation with Christopher's parents, his teachers and even the school administrators regarding intervention planning for Christopher. What would be the goal of these consultation sessions? Role play how you could engage in consultation with each of these groups. (**D2**)
4. What type of information should the school psychologist provide to the teachers regarding how best to handle Christopher in the classroom? What types of information is it appropriate to share to ensure that they don't inadvertently escalate similar situations as they occur? (**D2, O4**)
5. Research some of the best practices and controversies/concerns regarding policing in schools. What are best practices for involving school resource officers in situations such as the one described in this case? What are the potential problems and how can they be managed? (**O4**)
6. Review Huberty's (2014) *Best Practices in School-Based Interventions for Anxiety and Depression* and apply the relevant elements to this case. What would you recommend be done to assist Christopher based on your review of this chapter?

Case Three: Class-Wide Consultation

Ms. Carter is an enthusiastic teacher in her second year of teaching. During her first year as a teacher, she was assigned to teach in fifth grade. However, due to increasing enrollment for kindergarten, the school realized over the summer months the need to add another class of kindergarten this year and Ms. Carter was assigned in August to a kindergarten classroom. Given late registrations for kindergarten, unfortunately Ms. Carter was only given about two weeks' notice that she would be teaching kindergarten. Being an enthusiastic teacher, Ms. Carter jumped into planning by reviewing the kindergarten curriculum. However, given her focus on creating instructional materials for the kindergarten level, she did not really have time to change her class-wide behavior management plan prior to the beginning of school. She did her best to adapt the program that was successful during the previous year with her fifth graders to the kindergarten environment. It is now November and she has come into the school psychologist's office, Ms. Kay, in tears after school one day. She reported that she feels that she has "lost control" over the class, as the students had yet to adjust to the behavioral expectations of kindergarten. Ms. Kay agreed to conduct some classroom observations and Ms. Carter indicated her willingness to work with the school psychologist to try to improve some of the behavior management and classroom procedures in the class.

The school psychologist, Ms. Kay, observed the class on four different occasions throughout the morning activities (morning circle time, rotations to stations, and during independent work time) for 60 minutes in total during each observation. Ms. Kay tracked behavioral concerns of multiple students (18 students total) in the classroom (see Table 4.1). During these observations she noted occasions of calling out behaviors, non-compliance with directions and potential safety concerns (i.e., children running in the classroom with scissors, students shoving one another to get a preferred spot in one of the stations). Further, when analyzing the classroom environment, the school psychologist found that the children did not seem to understand the classroom procedures, the stated rules of the classroom, and the behavior management system in use. Ms. Kay noticed that the procedures and classroom rules were written in complex, multi-step language, which might be confusing for kindergarten students. The focus on writing the rules out rather than using pictures and more appealing graphics also seemed to Ms. Kay to be developmentally inappropriate for the kindergarten level. Ms. Kay also noticed that the classroom space was quite cluttered, both on the walls and in the actual physical space. With extra desks and furniture, Ms. Kay noticed that the children did not have a lot of space to move around the room comfortably. It was also noted that all the classroom materials (scissors, markers, crayons, etc.) were out on desks and tables for all children to access at any time.

Ms. Kay and Ms. Carter met to review the data collected by the school psychologist during the four observations and agreed to prioritize the safety concerns (running in class, pushing other students). While they are concerned with all the problematic behaviors occurring within the class, the safety concerns were prioritized given the risk of harm to the students. They discussed making global changes to all the classroom rules and procedures, reorganizing the classroom space, streamlining the rules to focus on the prioritized

Table 4.1 Class Behavior Observation Data

Baseline	Calling Out	Inability to Follow Directions	Safety Concerns (running with items, pushing/ shoving)
Observation 1	14	11	11
Observation 2	15	9	12
Observation 3	18	14	9
Observation 4	16	13	12
Intervention Phase			
Observation 1	13	11	7
Observation 2	11	10	5
Observation 3	12	9	6
Observation 4	11	7	7
Observation 5	10	7	5
Observation 6	11	8	4
Observation 7	10	5	2
Observation 8	12	3	3
Observation 9	14	2	1
Observation 10	14	2	1

issues, and implementing a positive behavior reward system. Ms. Kay agrees to assist with continued weekly observations to determine the effectiveness of the new procedures and interventions put into place. Table 4.1 and Figure 4.1 include the data from the baseline and intervention phases.

Discussion Questions

1. Ms. Kay and Ms. Carter decided to focus on safety concerns as the target of intervention. Do you agree with this decision based on the baseline data collected? Why or why not? (**D1**)

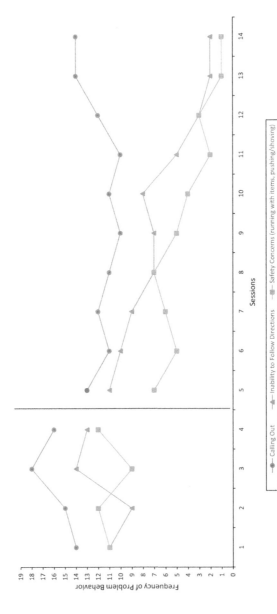

Figure 4.1 Class-Wide Intervention Data

2. How might Ms. Kay and Ms. Carter better operationalize the behaviors of concern (safety concerns, inability to follow directions, calling out)? Write out operationalized definitions for each of these categories. (**D4**)

3. Upon reviewing the progress monitoring data, are the interventions put into place working? Why or why not? (**D1**)

4. What might you suggest next in this case? What should be prioritized and why? (**D4**)

5. Ms. Carter was open to suggestions to assist her behavior management in class as she seemed to realize that she needed some assistance with updating her classroom procedures/management to younger grades. How did her openness to consultation with Ms. Kay influence the outcomes in this case? How might this case have proceeded differently if Ms. Carter was not open to making changes to her classroom management/procedures? (**D2**)

Advanced Applications

1. During this class-wide intervention, Ms. Kay has been conducting the weekly observations to determine the effectiveness of the interventions. She comes to the class for 60 minutes each week to collect the data in all categories. This may not be feasible for all school psychologists. Design a more stream-lined data collection plan that still allows for data collection for progress monitoring. (**D1**)

2. The interventions put into place in this classroom were designed to update classroom management/procedures so that they work better with younger children. Thus, the intervention plan was quite general. If more specific interventions were needed, research some possible evidence-based interventions that could be utilized in this class for the identified areas of concern. (**D4**)

3. This data represents whole-class data. Suppose that the analyses of data find that the continued calling out behavior is mostly from one child in the class who has not adapted to the classroom routine. If the majority of the continued calling out is from this one child, what individual intervention might be suggested to change this behavior? How could this intervention for one child be monitored? (**D4**)

4. How can the school psychologist ensure that the school administration sees value in her participation in class-wide interventions such as the one described? What data should be presented to document that this is an effective use of the school psychologist's time? (**O1, O3, O4**)

Case Four: When the Pandemic Came Along

Jason is an 8th-grade, White male student who attends John F. Kennedy (JFK) Middle School. Jason is described as an average student and teachers have reported in the past to his parents that he seems socially withdrawn, at times unmotivated, and is difficult to engage with when teachers attempt to have conversations with him. He is generally quiet in class and does not seek out interactions with teachers, even when he needs assistance with an assignment. He has historically received Bs and Cs in his academic courses. Jason's mother indicates that he is quiet and shy kid who she describes as "socially awkward." He does have a few friends who he talks with at school, although they live on the opposite sides of town, so they do not often get together after school or on the weekends. Jason is not involved in sports or any other extra-curricular activities. His mother reports that he spends most of his free time in the basement playing video games.

When the pandemic began in March of his eighth-grade year, JFK Middle School, like most middle schools, switched to virtual learning. The school did not reopen again for the remainder of the school year. Almost immediately, Jason's teachers reported concerns that Jason was not logging-in to their virtual class sessions and that he was only infrequently submitting assignments. When the school psychologist reached out to the family in May of that year due to his now failing grades in most academic classes, Jason's mother reported that she was becoming increasingly concerned about Jason. She reported that he was extremely unmotivated to complete any academic work. His mother was a nurse and essential worker during the pandemic; therefore, she is not always home during virtual instruction to monitor Jason's attendance. She reported that she would come home from work to find that Jason had slept until the afternoon and then played video games for the remainder of the afternoon. His mother reported that he was not communicating with any friends and she feared that he was playing video games with people that he had only met through the gaming world. She was also concerned because Jason's father, who he would typically see every other weekend, was now not visiting due to his own concerns about the virus because of his ongoing health concerns. As an only child, Jason's mother fears that he is spending too much time alone and asks the school psychologist for suggestions of how she can help her son to cope with the social isolation and withdrawal that she is witnessing from him.

The school psychologist, Ms. Nguyen, was a bit intimidated by this request, not sure how to help a student, teacher, or parent in these stressful and uncertain times. She decided to consult the APA *Guidelines for Practice of Telepsychology* (2013) and the growing body of research supporting tele-consultation to see what models existed that she might use to guide her next steps. She was interested to find that there were studies confirming teacher's acceptability of teleconsultation (Fischer, Dart et al., 2016; Fischer, Dart, Radley et al., 2016.; Schultz et al., 2017), consistency with or improvements upon face-to-face methods (Fischer et al., 2017), and positive student outcomes (e.g., Bice-Urbach & Kratochwill, 2016; Fischer, Dart, Radley et al., 2016). Ms. Nguyen viewed the APA Division 16 webinar, which was recorded and available free online (see Fischer, 2020). She stumbled across two journal special issues that focused solely on the topic of teleconsultation, *The Journal of Educational and Psychological Consultation* volume 28, number three (2018) and the *Journal of Behavioral Education* volume 29 (2020). She found the introduction articles by Fischer and his colleagues (2018), Bice-Urbach et al. (2018), and Rispoli and Machalicek (2020) to be important overview resources for the advances in telehealth in education. Armed with that information and recognizing her own efficacy in delivering face-to-face consultation services, she felt ready to try teleconsultation.

Discussion Questions

1. Jason is clearly struggling with virtual learning during the pandemic. Name some ways that the school could have been more proactive early on in offering support to Jason and his family. (**D3, D4, D7**)
2. Why was it important for Ms. Nguyen to consult the relevant literature and research around teleconsultation? (**D9**)
3. What hypotheses do you have regarding Jason's academic performance during virtual instruction? How are Jason's academic and social/emotional concerns related? (**D3, D4**)
4. Jason is referred to as unmotivated throughout this case. What may be a more positive conceptualization of the areas of concern? (**D4**)
5. While the switch to virtual instruction seems to have negatively impacted Jason's grades and is the trigger that caused the school to reach out to Jason's mother, there is some evidence to suggest that Jason may have needed additional support from the school prior to this. What are some suggestions for earlier interventions and/or supports that could have been put in place or at least explored during Jason's earlier elementary/middle school years? (**D3, D4**)
6. Now that Ms. Nguyen is ready to offer teleconsultation, who should be her consultee? Why? (**D2**)

Advanced Applications

1. Review some of the references that Ms. Nguyen initially consulted about teleconsultation. Using that information, how might you approach tele-consultation for this case? What steps would you take? What practical and legal considerations would be needed? (**D2, D10**)

2. Design an assessment plan to better understand some of Jason's particu-lar needs. (**D1**)

3. Research and design an intervention plan to provide support to Jason and his mother. (**D3, D4, D7, D9**)

4. The pandemic completely upended the educational system in the entire country. What were some of the immediate and long-term negative impacts of the pandemic on students' learning? How about on stu-dents' mental health? How should schools continue to respond to these impacts? (**D5**)

5. Some believe that one of the positive side effects of the pandemic might be the reimagination of how we educate our children, which has not been critically changed in generations. One example includes an increase in investment in technology-based education that may have benefits for children long after the pandemic has ended. How might this be a long-term benefit? What are the potential drawbacks of an over-reliance on technology-based education? What are other potential positive long-term outcomes may emerge regarding how we educate children in this country? (**D5, O1, O2**)

6. What additional professional development, specific to school psycholo-gists, might need to happen to ensure that they have the skills to support children during this pandemic? (**O6**)

References

American Psychological Association. (2013). Guidelines for the practice of telepsychology. *American Psychologist, 68*, 791–800. https://doi.org/10.1037/a0035001

Bice-Urbach, B. J., & Kratochwill, T. R. (2016). Teleconsultation: The use of technology to improve evidence-based practices in rural communities. *Journal of School Psychology, 56*, 27–43. https://doi.org/10.1016/j.jsp.2016.02.001

Bice-Urbach, B. J., Kratochwill, T. R., & Fischer, A. J. (2018). Teleconsultation: Application to provision of consultation services for school consultants. *Journal of Educational and Psychological Consultation, 28*(3), 1–24. https://doi.org/10.1080/10474412.2017.1389651

Fischer, A. J. (2020, May 8). *How to school psych during a global pandemic: Supporting students through teleconsultation with caregivers and educators.* [Webinar]. http://apadivision16.

org/2020/05/webinar-recording-for-how-to-school-psych-during-a-global-pandemic-supporting-students-through-teleconsultation-with-caregivers-and-educators/

Fischer, A. J., Collier-Meek, M. A., Bloomfield, B., Erchul, W. P., & Gresham, F. M. (2017). A comparison of problem identification interviews conducted face-to-face and via videoconferencing using the consultation analysis record. *Journal of School Psychology, 63,* 63–76. https://doi.org/10.1016/j.jsp.2017.03.009

Fischer, A. J., Dart, E. H., Leblanc, H., Hartman, K. L., Steeves, R. O., & Gresham, F. M. (2016). An investigation of the acceptability of videoconferencing within a school-based behavioral consultation framework. *Psychology in the Schools, 53*(3), 240–252. https://doi.org/10.1002/pits.21900

Fischer, A. J., Dart, E. H., Radley, K. C., Richardson, D., Clark, R., & Wimberly, J. (2016). An evaluation of the effectiveness and acceptability of teleconsultation. *Journal of Educational and Psychological Consultation. 27*(4), 437–458. www.tandfonline.com/doi/full/10.1080/10474412.2016.1235978

Fischer, A. J., Erchul, W. P., & Schultz, B. K. (2018). Teleconsultation as the new frontier of educational and psychological consultation: Introduction to the special issue. *Journal of Educational and Psychological Consultation, 28*(3), 249–254. https://doi.org/10.1080/10474412.2018.1425880

Herbstrith, J. C., & Tobin, R. M. (2014). Best practices in group counseling. In P. L. Harrison & A. Thomas (Eds.), *Best practices in school psychology: Student-level services* (pp. 305–320). National Association of School Psychologists.

Huberty, T. J. (2014). Best practices in school-based interventions for anxiety and depression. In P. L. Harrison & A. Thomas (Eds.), *Best practices in school psychology* (pp. 349–364). National Association of School Psychologists.

National Association of School Psychology. (2020). *The professional standards of the national association of school psychologists.* National Association of School Psychologists.

Pas, E. T., Kaiser, L., Rabinowitz, J. A., Lochman, J. E., & Bradshaw, C. P. (2020). Identifying factors associated with patterns of student attendance and participation in a group Tier 2 preventive intervention: Implications for adaptation, *Journal of Applied School Psychology, 36*(2), 198–226. https://doi.org/10.1080/15377903.2020.1714860

Rispoli, M., & Machalicek, W. (2020). Advances in telehealth and behavioral assessment and intervention in education: Introduction to the special issue. *Journal of Behavioral Education, 29*(2), 189–194. https://doi.org/10.1007/s10864-020-09383-5

Schultz, B. K., Zoder-Martell, K. A., Fischer, A., Collier-Meek, M. A., Erchul, W. P., & Schoermann, A. M. (2017). When is teleconsultation acceptable to school psychologists? *Journal of Educational and Psychological Consultation, 28*(3), 279–296. https://doi.org/10.1080/10474412.2017.1385397

Understanding School-Wide Practices to Promote Learning

5

Domain 5: School-Wide Practices to Promote Learning

"School psychologists understand systems structures, organization, and theory; general and special education programming; implementation science; and evidence-based, school-wide practices that promote learning, positive behavior, and mental health. School psychologists, in collaboration with others, develop and implement practices and strategies to create and maintain safe, effective, and supportive learning environments for students and school staff." (NASP, 2020, p. 6)

One of the vital roles that school psychologists can play is at the school-wide or system-level. With the expertise and knowledge that school psychologists have gained through their training, they can and should be integral to school-wide problem-solving to support the behavior, mental health, and academic development of all children. The cases within this chapter demonstrate some of this wide variety of ways that school psychologists might be involved with school-wide practices to promote learning. The cases all focus on different school-wide practices that directly impact student success.

Whether through participating in program development and design, program evaluation, the professional development of teachers and other staff in the school, or the monitoring of program implementation and success, school psychologists have the skills to truly make a difference in the school organization to positively benefit children. While using collaborative communication and problem-solving skills, school psychologists can make a difference by understanding how teams and schools as organizations function, how to establish effective collaborative problem-solving units within schools, how to engage multiple stakeholders for common goals, and how to provide professional development and ongoing support to staff and families. Cases one and two provide examples of this in practice, with a focus on the PBIS model and MTSS processes, respectively, in schools. These cases provide sample data for analysis and discussion, specifically related to how to improve the process and ensure ongoing consistency in implementation.

School psychologists also can and should be involved in the development and ongoing evaluation of school improvement plans and/or strategic development goals for schools. They might offer their expertise in the design and delivery of needs assessment for various stakeholder groups or in the recommendations of various evidence-based programs or practices to foster development based on individual school/community needs. To foster discussion about these important skills, Case Four provides an example of how a school psychologist might be involved in the design of a needs assessment and the use of that data to make suggestions for improving school psychologists' professional development opportunities.

School psychologists might become involved with a wide range of school-based programs, including programs foster positive school climate, programs that develop tiered systems of support for children's academic development, programs that increase school attendance, programs that reduce bullying, programs that use positive behavioral support to recognize students' successes, and many more. School psychologists can also be involved in the selection and utilization of various screening measures to better understand the students in the school who may need more academic, social/emotional, or behavioral support. The third case focuses on data-based decision-making for school-wide programs with a scenario involving how a school might analyze and effectively utilize data from a universal screener related to diversity and school climate.

According to NASP (2020, p. 7), "school psychologists analyze systems-level problems and identify factors that influence learning and behavior. . . . They help other school leaders evaluate outcomes . . . support shared decision-making practices . . . and meet general public accountability responsibilities." Cases One and Three provide opportunities to look at potential equity issues that exist within a school. This allows for discussion of the school psychologist's role in analyzing and sharing that data for accountability and team problem-solving.

Case One: Beyond Token Rewards: Ensuring Ongoing Improvement With PBIS Implementation

The staff at Ocean Air Elementary school were committed to student success. They recently engaged in a school-wide overhaul of their discipline system. They decided to adopt School-Wide Positive Behavior Support (SWPBS, Sugai & Horner, 2002). A core group of committed teachers and staff attended the SWBPS Team training three years ago and started to implement SWPBS school-wide that year. They worked very hard in the first year to ramp up their school store to include many more rewards and incentives that students could "purchase" with their "Dolphin Dollars." A Dolphin Dollar was a token that students received when they were "caught being good," which meant displaying one of the school's core values (e.g., Respectful, Responsible, Safe). The SWPBS Team also worked hard that year to develop school-wide activities and events that students could attend weekly on "Fun Friday," if they earned enough points for the week (e.g., a Dolphin Dance or Dolphins & Donuts). The team was very excited to see the impact of the activities that they had developed and how much the students enjoyed the new incentives.

Each year, the SWPBS Team receives evaluation feedback from the school district's SWPBS Coordinator. The coordinator used the SWPBS School Evaluation Tool (SET, Horner et al., 2004) evaluation to collect data and provide feedback on SWPBS fidelity. In the third year, the team was proud of their progress each year, but dismayed to see that they were still just short of the 80 percent benchmark to be considered a high implementing team. Their overall SET score was 78 percent. They reviewed the graph of their progress over the past three years (see Figure 5.1). Their highest feature and most notable growth were in their ongoing systems for rewarding behavioral expectations, with a score of 85 percent. The coordinator noted their consistent use of the Dolphin Dollar system. The coordinator indicated that when interviewed, some staff members felt the Dolphin Dollar system was not effective because they felt like they were just "bribing students to behave."

In terms of behavioral expectation definition, the team received a score of 52 percent. The feedback indicated that they did have three positively stated expectations but noted that these were not prominently displayed in all classrooms, hallways, or special areas. In some cases, the expectations that were posted were slightly different than what the team indicated they should

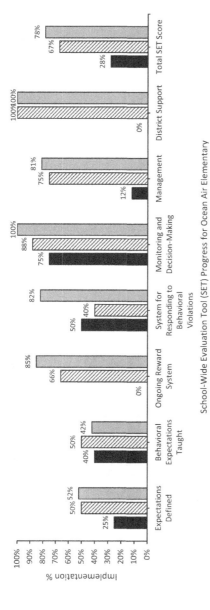

School-Wide Evaluation Tool (SET) Progress for Ocean Air Elementary

Figure 5.1 School-Wide Evaluation Tool (SET) Progress for Ocean Air Elementary Year

be (e.g., not Respectful, Responsible, Safe; instead, the 4 Bs "Be Ready, Be Respectful, Be Proud, Be You!"). Additionally, the team earned 42 percent for the "behavior expectations taught" feature. The coordinator indicated in the feedback that there was nothing in writing to teach students the behavior expectations (e.g., no lesson plans for what it means to be respectful, responsible, or safe in the cafeteria or on the playground). When interviewed, only 65 percent of the staff agreed that they had taught or reinforced the three behavioral expectations this year, and only 30 percent of the teachers and students could recite those expectations.

The team also noted their progress in recent years for responding to behavioral violations, which went up from 40–50 percent to 82 percent. They felt particularly proud of how they cleaned up and clarified their office discipline referral process for student behavior infractions. The staff now knew the difference between a major and a minor referral and were more consistently using the referral form to document concerns. However, a review of their triangle data (see Figure 5.2) from the School-wide Information System (SWIS, SWIS Suite, 2020) indicated that they had a few students who were "highflyers," meaning that they received most of the office discipline referrals for

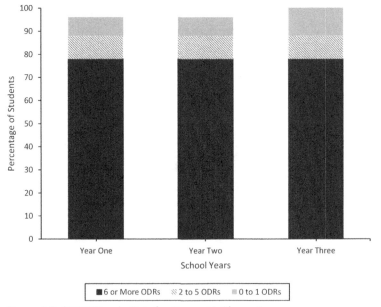

Figure 5.2 SWIS Triangle Data for Ocean Air Elementary

Table 5.1 Analysis of Repeat Office Referrals by Race/Ethnicity at Ocean Air Elementary

Ethnicity	# of Students Enrolled	# Students With Referrals	% of Students Within Ethnicity With Referrals	Risk Index
American Indian/Alaskan Native	8	4	50%	0.50
Asian	8	1	12.5%	.12
Hispanic/Latino	97	37	38.14%	.38
Black	70	55	78.57%	.79
White	302	99	32.78%	.33
Pacific Islander/ Native Hawaiian	3	0	0%	.00
Multiracial	24	3	12.5%	.13
Totals	**512**	**199**		

behavioral violations. These students were not allowed to participate in the "Fun Friday" activities if they had office referrals for the week or if they didn't earn enough Dolphin Dollars. The coordinator provided feedback that the school should analyze their data to determine who made up this group of repeated referrals. Upon analysis, the school identified the following students as those with the most frequent referrals (Table 5.1). They compared that data to their school demographics to try to determine if any equity issues existed and to develop their action plan for the next school year.

Discussion Questions

1. After reviewing all of the data presented, what is working well in this school? What needs to be improved? (**D1, D5**)
2. What is the school psychologist's role in working with this team to analyze this type of fidelity or equity data? A school psychologist was not mentioned in the case. Should they be part of the team? Why or why not? (**D1, D8, D5, D10**)

3. If you were a member of this team, what areas would you recommend prioritizing in the school's action plan? (**D1, D5**)
4. What types of services would you recommend for the areas of prioritized need? (**D5, D6**)
5. Based on the data in Table 5.1, what were the demographics of the students who were receiving repeat office referrals? In other words, who was excluded from the rewards and incentives? How might the school psychologist help the school analyze and address this to provide more culturally responsive PBIS? (**D1, D8**)

Advanced Applications

1. After more exploration, you notice that most repeat referrals are coming from one or two classrooms. Role play a conversation with one of the teachers to discuss this concern and offer consultation or coaching services. (**D2**)
2. Assuming that the teachers in the scenario are interested in engaging in consultation about their classroom management, what would be your first steps in establishing the consultation relationship? What model would you follow and why? (**D2**)
3. Imagine that you are a part of this PBIS Team Meeting. Upon reviewing this data, develop an action plan. Include a measurable goal for the year and activities to support that goal. (**D2, D5**)

Case Two: Comparing Standard Protocol and Problem-Solving Approaches

At Cross Town Elementary School, the school psychologist, Mr. Beery, was a member of the school's MTSS Team. The team noticed that there was a group of third-grade students in need of "strategic" intervention. This meant that the students scored in the "at-risk" range on their benchmark fluency assessments. They were then assigned to receive Tier II reading intervention. At this school, that meant that the students would be placed in a reading intervention group, with the reading specialist, who implemented the Read Naturally® (Read Naturally®, 2020) program 30 minutes daily during intervention block. The students received the intervention from October through January. All students made progress via the DIBELS Oral Reading Fluency (ORF, UO DIBELS®, n.d.) probes from October to January (see Figure 5.3).

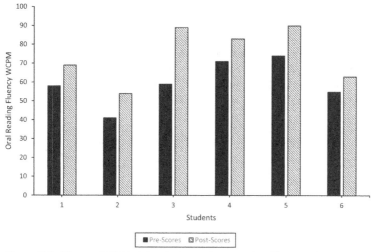

Figure 5.3 "Strategic" Third-Grade Group Intervention Fluency Progress

The MTSS Team focused solely on helping the kids on "the bubble" receive the strategic small group services. This meant that there were still a few students in third grade who scored lower on the fluency benchmark but did not receive the Tier II intervention because they appeared to be in an "intensive range." This left their teacher, Ms. Applegate, perplexed about how to best meet their needs. She requested support from Mr. Beery for those students. Mr. Beery offered his consultation services to Ms. Applegate. Together, from October to November, they worked through a problem-solving process in the problem-identification and analysis phase to better understand the students' reading concerns. They did informal curriculum-based assessment with one of the students from her class that was scoring in the intensive range on the fluency assessments. They assessed the student in terms of word recognition, phonics, fluency, and comprehension.

In analyzing the data, it appeared that the student read slowly when he came to an unknown word. He spent a long time trying to break larger multisyllabic words apart. With this information, they identified advanced decoding as the prioritized area of concern because they hypothesized that his labored and inaccurate decoding of multisyllabic words hindered his fluency. Together, they developed a classroom-based intervention to help the student learn ways to decode multisyllabic words. They utilized an evidence-based intervention that was easy to use in the classroom without specialized training or curriculum, the phoneme-grapheme mapping strategy (Earle & Sayeski, 2016) in addition to fluency practice via repeated reading

(Evidence Based Intervention Network, 2011; Zimmerman & Reed, 2019) of instructional level text that included the target multisyllabic words. The teacher implemented the strategies with the target student, but also with a group of the other students that had similar decoding and fluency needs. The target student in that group made fluency gains rapidly (see Figure 5.4). All the students in the instructional consultation group improved their fluency quickly (Figure 5.5). In fact, the teacher consultation group

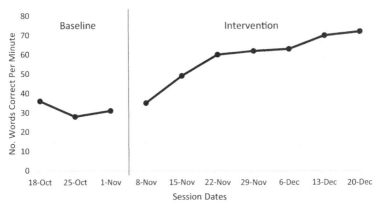

Figure 5.4 "Intensive" Third-Grade Student Intervention Progress: Decoding Intervention, Fluency Gains

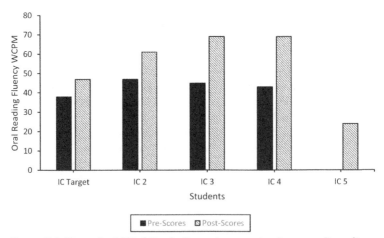

Figure 5.5 "Intensive" Third-Grade Group Intervention Progress: Decoding Intervention, Fluency Gains

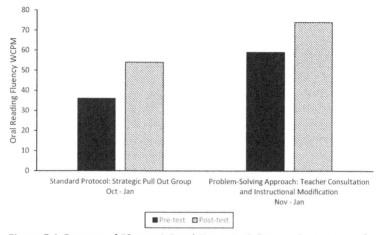

Figure 5.6 Progress of "Strategic" and "Intensive" Groups: Comparison of Standard Protocol Approach and Problem-Solving Approach

made more progress than the Tier II pull-out group in less time because they were further behind and Ms. Applegate and Mr. Beery took an additional month to conduct the problem-identification/analysis stage before intervening (see Figure 5.6).

Discussion Questions

1. What is the school psychologist's role in working with a school-wide MTSS team? What were the benefits of Mr. Beery's involvement with this team? (**D1, D2, D3, D5, D10**)
2. Why might this group of students have progressed more rapidly than the students receiving the Tier II intervention? What could this mean in terms of improvements needed in the Tier II intervention stage? (**D1, D5**)
3. What were some of the limitations of this MTSS Team's approach to problem-solving? What might have happened if Mr. Beery was not involved in offering consultative services? (**D1, D2, D3, D9**)
4. In looking at the outcomes for this case, is it appropriate to call the groups or students, "intensive" and "strategic" after all? Why or why not? (**D8, D10**)

Advanced Applications

1. Read and discuss Erchul's (2011) *School Consultation and Response to Intervention: A Tale of Two Literatures* in relation to this case. Compare and contrast the advantages and disadvantages to both approaches, the Standard Protocol Approach the MTSS Team took for the Tier II "Strategic" group, as compared to the Problem-Solving Approach used with the teacher for the "Intensive" group. How might school-wide practices need to take both into account when building team structures and processes? (**D3, D5**)

2. Research the evidence base for Read Naturally (Institute of Education Sciences, n.d.). What reading skills are the most likely to improve using this intervention? (**D3, D9**)

3. Review the concept of the skill-by-treatment interaction (Burns et al., 2014) to describe why each intervention may have been the best fit for each group. What might have happened if the students in Ms. Applegate's group been placed in the fluency intervention program? Would they have made progress as quickly? What is your hypothesis based on the skill-by-treatment interaction concept? (**D3**)

4. What assessments would you have conducted if you were the school psychologist and consultant for this case, to better understand the students' reading skills and needs? (**D1, D3**)

5. Review the phoneme-grapheme mapping intervention (e.g., Earle & Sayeski, 2016). Create an intervention script and fidelity checklist to use to consult with a teacher like Ms. Applegate to implement a similar strategy. (**D2, D3**)

Case Three: School Diversity Climate Assessment and Intervention

Dr. Williams, a well-established veteran school psychologist, recently switched to a new school in her district, Lakeside Elementary, a diverse Title 1 suburban elementary school (see Table 5.2). She immediately recognized the mismatch in terms of racial, ethnic, and socio-economic status between the staff and the students at the school. She wanted to learn more about the perspectives from various stakeholders in the school. In the first few weeks of working at this school, she made it a point to introduce herself to the Black Student Achievement Program (BSAP) Liaison, Mrs. Jackson, and the Hispanic Association (HA) Liaison, Ms. Benita. Ms. Williams was pleased to see that there were affinity groups and resources established within the

Table 5.2 Demographics of Lakeside Elementary

	Staff	Students
American Indian/Alaskan	0%	<5%
Asian	0%	10.5%
Black	8%	51.6%
Hawaiian/Pacific Islander	0%	<5%
Hispanic/Latino	5%	25.4%
White	83%	6.3%
Multiracial	4%	5.8%
Free and Reduced Meals	n/a	59.4%

school. She was troubled, however, to learn from Mrs. Jackson that the teachers attributed student learning or behavioral problems to the students' home lives and lack of parent support. Ms. Benita agreed and added that often the parents shy away from school events because they do not want to appear critical or rude by asking clarifying questions of the school or teachers.

Ms. Williams was pleased with the school environment. Unlike her previous school, she noted that it was clean, safe, and free of vandalism, defacement, and broken objects. Additionally, many areas had school logos, which helps to promote a sense of school community and school ownership. Adults were also present in these areas, especially during high traffic times, which promoted student-teacher interactions and teacher-parent interactions, during pick-up and drop-off. She particularly liked the sense of cultural pride visible in the school, with the prominent display of pennants from Historically Black Colleges and Universities, as well as photographs and biographies of famous Black and Latino Americans. She noticed that this was only seen in the wing near the back of the school where the BSAP and HA liaisons had their offices. The front hallway and wing of the school were more sparsely decorated with a photo of the current President of the United States, the governor of the state, and the school superintendent, all white males. There were photos of the past student government leaders of the school and current students of the month. Ms. Williams noticed that the students in those photos were disproportionately white, especially given the school's demographics.

As Ms. Williams got more acclimated in the school, she noticed that there were several school events to attempt to build a sense of community. These

Table 5.3 School Climate Survey Data

Student Engagement	63%
Employee Engagement	60%
Student Hope	43%

community events were monthly and were planned by each liaison for their respective group of families. Mrs. Jackson hosted a "Soul-Food Potluck" for the BSAP families to highlight their favorite dishes. Ms. Benita planned a "Bilingual Family Literacy Night," filled with family reading games and activities in both English and Spanish. A small handful of dedicated teachers attended these family community events. There were also PTA meetings, which typically had higher teacher attendance, and were planned by the PTA Board. The PTA Board primarily consisted of white female parents.

Ms. Williams was increasingly interested in understanding the climate and culture of the school, so she looked up climate survey data that were available for each school in her district, on the district's website. She noticed that overall student and staff perceptions of their engagement were not impressive, ranging from 60–63 percent (see Table 5.3). She was most struck, but the low rating of hope by students in the school (43 percent). She noticed the ratings that were particularly low were "I have a mentor who encourages my development" and "I can find many ways around problems."

To continue her comprehensive appraisal of the school climate and culture, Ms. Williams started looking up more data on enrollment or eligibility patterns across the school. She noticed that there were patterns of over and underrepresentation that were also concerning (see Table 5.4). The representation patterns of students within groups appeared to maintain racial or ethnic stereotypes. She could also see clear indications that students who lacked financial resources were also missing out on important opportunities such as extracurricular sports or science clubs. She contemplated sharing her observation of some of the needs and issues with the administrator of the school but was unsure of how or where to start.

Discussion Questions

1. What is the school psychologists' role regarding exploring the diversity and climate issues as seen in this case? What are ethical and legal considerations? (**D5, D8, D10**)

Table 5.4 School Participation by Race/Ethnicity

	% Enrolled	% in Sports	% in Student Government	% in Gifted	% in Science Club
American Indian/Alaskan	<5%	<5%	0%	0%	0%
Asian	10.5%	<5%	15%	30%	40%
Black	51.6%	70%	15%	10%	<5%
Hawaiian/Pacific Islander	<5%	<5%	0%	0%	0%
Hispanic/Latinx	25.4%	10%	0%	10%	7%
White	6.3%	15%	70%	50%	50%
Multiracial	5.8%	3%	0%	0%	<5%
Free and Reduced Meals	59.4%	25%	0%	0%	0%

2. What are some of the protective and positive features of the school culture and climate? What are the concerning aspects? What would you prioritize as needs? Explain your rationale. (**D5, D6, D7, D8**)
3. What types of assessment activities have been important for Ms. Williams to conduct in her first months in the school? Why? What other assessment activities might you recommend for her to understand the school diversity culture and climate better? (**D1, D5, D8**)
4. Ms. Williams appears to be doing much of this work alone. How could she enlist the support of others to do this work with her? Why might it be important to include others? (**D2, D5, D8**)

Advanced Applications

1. Research and list specific school culture and climate tools that a school psychologist could use to analyze diversity and equity issues at the school-level. (**D1, D5, D8, D9**)
2. Review the literature on developing an equity team and best practices on how to facilitate needs assessment and school-wide intervention on diversity climate issues in a school. Develop a list of steps and strategies

that a school psychologist, who is in a similar position as Ms. Williams, could utilize to guide their work. (**D1, D2, D5, D7, D8, D9**)

3. Research and describe at least one evidence-based practice to address one of the issues you identified in this case. Provide rationale for why you selected this intervention. (**D5, D9**)

4. Role play a consultation session between Ms. Williams and the school principal to practice administrative consultation around an issue identified in this case. (**D2, D5, D8**)

Case Four: Prioritizing Time With Fellow School Psychologists: The Case for Specialized Programming

Stacey works as a school psychologist in a mid-size district in a suburban school district. She is busy in her day-to-day work as a school psychologist serving an elementary and middle school and often feels resentful when she is asked to give up time in her schools to attend various professional development sessions with other teachers and staff. After several years of feeling this way, she decides to begin speaking with other school psychologists in the district to see if they also feel the same way. In her conversations, she begins to realize that other school psychologists feel like her, but that it seems to be related to the type of professional development (PD) that is offered during these days, which are geared much more towards teachers. Stacey approaches the Supervisor of Special Services and asks if she can design and distribute a needs assessment to determine areas in which school psychologists feel they need additional PD and the supervisor agrees. Stacey has been out of graduate school for several years and therefore has limited experience/knowledge regarding best practices in needs assessment/survey development.

To ensure that she creates a well-designed survey, she researches best practices online, reads multiple articles about survey/needs assessment development and she collaborates with another school psychologist in the district who is currently enrolled in a doctoral program in school psychology and thus has more recent knowledge about survey design. After the survey is created, they send it to the twenty-eight school psychologists in the district electronically. To their pleasant surprise, there is great interest in completing the survey and they get a 95 percent return rate.

The results demonstrated that overwhelmingly school psychologists report a desire for professional development sessions to be designed specifically for their needs as school psychologists. In open-ended comments, a theme emerged that the school psychologists greatly value their time together during PD days, since in the day-to-day work as a school psychologist they do not have another school psychology professional in their school to collaborate and problem-solve with around pressing issues. As far as topics for professional development, 70 percent indicated their greatest need is related to academic-based interventions and a need to have a better understanding of evidence-based academic interventions. After this category, the next largest need was for school-wide SEL programs (20 percent indicated this as their top priority), while 10 percent of respondents indicated various other priorities (new standardized assessment training when they are released, best practices in threat assessment).

Based on these results, the supervisor of special services designed the next full-day professional development session to include a presentation on evidence-based academic interventions followed by one hour of small-group processing of pressing issues/case presentations. The entire day was a success with participants indicating that they would turnkey the information presented about academic-based interventions back to their school-based teams. Further, the informal round-table discussion of cases was highly valued by participants who indicated that they greatly appreciated the opportunity to have informal conversations with other school psychologists. Arguably, the informal discussions and case presentations were viewed as the most valuable portion of this professional development day. The school psychologists spoke informally at the end of the day about ways that they can create more opportunities for collaboration, mentoring, case sharing, and general discussions about school psychology practice.

Discussion Questions

1. School psychologists often report that general PD sessions are not particularly helpful to them. What are the advantages and disadvantages of having various professionals come together for PD as an entire building? (O4, O5)

2. Stacey was motivated to create a needs assessment for distribution to her fellow school psychologists but understands that she may have limited or outdated information about best practices in survey design. Why was it important that she consulted the professional literature and other professionals in the school to ensure that she created a sound survey? What could be the consequences of a poorly designed needs assessment? (O5)

3. In this case, Stacey purposefully seeks out guidance from a colleague who is currently attending a doctoral program to ensure that they design

a needs assessment that is in keeping with the latest research on survey design. In what ways are collaboration between Universities (faculty and students) and K-12 schools crucial to reducing the "research to practice gap" that is often viewed as a problem in schools. (**D9, D10**)

4. What are possible reasons the school psychologists are so enthusiastic about increased opportunities for collaboration across the district? Why is it important for school psychologists to continue to collaborate with other practicing professionals? (**O5**)

Advanced Applications

1. What leadership opportunities are available for school psychologists who work in medium/large-size districts for developing programs to support the practice of school psychology? Provide ideas of how to develop programs and resources for school psychologists (PD opportunities, collaboration, case sharing/consultation, etc.). (**O5**)

2. The specific topic of this PD session was related to academic interventions. Design a plan for the participating school psychologists to turnkey this information back to their individual schools. What specific elements should be included in turnkey trainings to ensure success? What types of ongoing support might be needed to ensure that the new strategies for academic intervention design are incorporated into the practices of the staff at each school? (**D5**)

References

Burns, M. K., VanDerHeyden, A. M., & Zaslofsky, A. F. (2014). Best practices in delivering intensive academic interventions with a skill-by-treatment interaction. In P. L. Harrison & A. Thomas (Eds.), *Best practices in school psychology: Student-level services* (pp. 129–141). National Association of School Psychologists.

Earle, G. A., & Sayeski, K. L. (2016). Systematic instruction in phoneme-grapheme correspondence for students with reading disabilities. *Intervention in School and Clinic, 52*(5), 262–269. https://doi.org/10.1177/1053451216676798

Erchul, W. P. (2011). School consultation and response to intervention: A tale of two literatures. *Journal of Educational and Psychological Consultation, 21*(3), 191–208. https://doi.org/10.1080/10474412.2011.595198

Evidence Based Intervention Network. (2011, March 31). *Repeated readings.* Retrieved November 25, 2020, from https://ebi.missouri.edu/?p=79

Horner, R. H., Todd, A. W., & Lewis, T. (2004). The school-wide evaluation tool (SET): A research instrument for assessing school-wide positive behavior support. *Journal of Positive Behavior Interventions, 6*(1), 3–12. https://doi.org/10.1177/10983007040060010201

Institute of Education Sciences. (n.d.). *Read naturally®*. IES WWC What Works Clearinghouse. Retrieved November 25, 2020, from https://ies.ed.gov/ncee/wwc/Evidence Snapshot/407

National Association of School Psychology. (2020). *The professional standards of the national association of school psychologists*. National Association of School Psychologists.

Read Naturally®. (2020). *Read naturally®*. Retrieved November 25, 2020, from www.readnaturally.com/

Sugai, G., & Horner, R. (2002). The evolution of discipline practices: School-wide positive behavior supports. *Behavior Psychology in the Schools, 24*(1–2), 23–50.

SWIS Suite. (2020). *PBISApps*. Retrieved November 25, 2020, from www.pbisapps.org

UO DIBELS®. (n.d.). *DIBELS oral reading fluency and retell fluency (ORF)*. Retrieved November 25, 2020, from https://dibels.uoregon.edu/assessment/dibels/measures/orf.php

Zimmerman, L., & Reed, D. K. (2019, February 5). *Repeated reading with goal-setting for reading fluency: Reading quality rather than reading speed*. Iowa Reading Research Center. Retrieved November 25, 2020, from https://iowareadingresearch.org/blog/repeated-reading-fluency

Understanding Services to Promote Safe and Supportive Schools

6

Domain 6: Services to Promote Safe and Supportive Schools

"School psychologists understand principles and research related to social-emotional well-being, resilience and risk factors in learning, mental and behavioral health, services in schools and communities to support multitiered prevention and health promotion, and evidence-based strategies for creating safe and supportive schools. School psychologists, in collaboration with others, promote preventive and responsive services that enhance learning, mental and behavioral health, and psychological and physical safety and implement effective crisis prevention, protection, mitigation, response, and recovery." (NASP, 2020, p. 7)

One of the critical roles of school psychologists is their active participation in a wide array of services that ensure that schools are both safe and supportive to all children. This begins with understanding, evaluating, and participating in programs that foster a positive school climate with the goals of creating positive relationships among staff, families, and students in the school. School psychologists can be vital in ensuring that school and

community-wide programs are in place that specifically foster these positive relationships and help all students feel connected to school. School psychologists can also address systemic problems that can lead to problems in
the school and community environment, such as substance abuse, bullying,
self-harm, chronic absenteeism, and criminal behaviors. The fourth case
in this chapter focuses on the critical importance of continual evaluation
of the school climate and its role in prevention. In this case, there is an
opportunity for discussion of how schools can respond to data that suggests
issues in the school climate that might negatively impact the school as well
as individual students.

School psychologists should seek out opportunities to be involved in
decision-making as it relates to ensuring safe and supportive school environments. This might include evaluating the specific vulnerabilities and risks
that the school, district, and community may face to ensure that preventative programming and activities are in place, as well as procedures to react
to and mitigate the effect of various crises that may occur. Further, this
involves understanding and evaluating any early indicators of risks and the
implementation of comprehensive plans to conduct suicide risk and threat
assessments. Cases Two and Three, respectively, focus on threat assessment
and suicide prevention and allow for discussion of how schools can improve
these processes.

School psychologists also participate as key members of school safety
and school crisis teams, and assist in the prevention, protection, mitigation,
response, and recovery efforts of various types of crises. Case One highlights
the vital role of school safety and school crisis teams, with a specific focus on
the immediate and long-term responses needed after a major hurricane dev-
astates a community. School psychologists can also train teachers, administrators, and other staff in crisis prevention and intervention techniques to ensure
that all school staff are aware of how to create positive and safe environments
for all children.

The prevention and intervention strategies used by school psychologists related to establishing safe and secure school environments are broad.
School psychologists must have the skills and confidence to both prevent and
respond to a variety of situations that can occur in both the school environment and in the community. The cases within this chapter attempt to focus
on distinct types of preventative and responsive roles that school psychologists might be a part of in schools. From the first case, which focuses on a
natural disaster and the wide-ranging impact on the entire community and
school, to the second and third cases which focus on the importance of react-
ing appropriately to potential threats and reports of suicidal ideation, the

cases demonstrate the wide range of situations that can confront a school psychologist.

Case One: A Once-in-a-Lifetime Storm

Simpson Elementary School has always had an active school safety team and a crisis response team. The teams meet at least quarterly to review their procedures and policies in place and both teams have several members who have been trained in NASP's PREPaRE curriculum and have read the accompanying text (Brock et al., 2016). The school safety team conducts a vulnerability assessment at least once per year, continually updates policies/procedures, and is responsible for the training of staff annually. They also evaluate school-based data on school climate, school connectedness, bullying, and discipline incidents to determine how to better serve the school community, prevent conflicts between students, and strengthen school connectedness. The school crisis response team meets regularly to review procedures for responding to crises, practice the response to various emergency situations via tabletop exercises, plan school-wide emergency protocols/drills, and attend ongoing training in crisis response. They also routinely present to all staff in the building to ensure that all are kept current on their school-specific crisis plans and procedures.

Last year in October, a major, category five hurricane hit the small coastal community, which includes Simpson Elementary School. The impact of the hurricane was devastating to the community. The immediate devastation included the loss of life for 12 individuals in the community, although none of those who perished in the hurricane were school-aged children. The flooding and high winds also caused extensive damage to the elementary school, the regional high school in the area and to most of the homes of the families who attend these schools. In fact, 45 percent of the students who attend Simpson Elementary School had their homes destroyed during the hurricane or had enough damage to their homes that the houses were deemed uninhabitable. Simpson Elementary School was flooded on the entire first level of the school. All paper student records were destroyed in the flooding and much of the computer equipment was damaged. The entire community was without electricity for between 14 and 25 days and most residents did not have Wi-Fi for several weeks, which severely limited the entire community's ability to communicate with one another. Many of the teachers and staff who work at Simpson Elementary School were also negatively impacted by the storm, with many teachers suffering a great deal of damage to their homes in the storm.

The students who attended Simpson Elementary School did not attend school for at least the first three weeks after the storm, and some students missed even more school than this. The school building could not be used for the remainder of that school year, so the school administrative team worked with other local communities to allow students to begin attending other schools. The destruction of all the papers in the school building led to many difficulties in ensuring students, particularly students with special needs and IEPs, had the appropriate educational services in place at their new, temporary schools. Further, some students who were displaced by the storm did not provide information about where they were living and what school they were attending. All told, six percent of students were not accounted for when school services resumed and efforts to contact families to see where they had moved and where their children were attending school were not successful.

The students from Simpson Elementary School ended up being sent to six different school buildings to complete the school year, since many of the schools who accepted students were limited in how many students that they could accept. While mental health support was available in each of these buildings to support students, there was a sense that some students needed additional support. Some of the children reportedly regressed in both their behavior and academic progress while at their new schools. The mental health professionals also reported that some students reported traumatic experiences both from the night of the storm, including having to evacuate from their house quickly as the storm surge rose, and in the weeks following the storm.

It is now the summer after the storm and the team from Simpson Elementary School is grateful that the school building has now been repaired and school is expected to reopen in September. Both the school safety team and the school crisis team are meeting regularly over the summer to prepare for the reopening of the school building. A major goal is to aid and support the students returning to their school who have not been living in the community since the storm. They are concerned that these students may feel disconnected from the school and the community. They estimate that 10 percent of the students at the school are still not living in their original homes and will be commuting to school from surrounding communities until they are able to move back into their homes. They also want to review their response to this community crisis and update procedures. The team is eager to provide as much support for the children and families in their school and are concerned that they might be overlooking ways that they should be providing support. They also realize that some of the teachers and other staff may need additional support in their return to school, given their own ongoing hardships as the result of losing their own homes and dealing with the consequences of the storm on their own lives.

Discussion Questions

1. The school safety and crisis teams at Simpson Elementary School were active, well-prepared teams; however, the significant impact of the hurricane on the entire community was overwhelming for all involved. Discuss how you would prioritize the school's response in the immediate aftermath of the storm. What tasks need to occur immediately? How would you triage the response? (**D6**)

2. What different types of traumatic responses might you expect from children from this elementary school? (**D4**)

3. How might the reactions vary depending upon proximity to the event, long-term family impact (i.e., family displacement), academic impacts, and the age of children? What sorts of mental health supports might be needed for these children? (**D4**)

4. In evaluating their response to this crisis, what parts of their response should they reflect upon? In what areas could the school have been better prepared? (**D6**)

5. What sort of support might be necessary for the school staff from Simpson Elementary School? (**D6**)

6. The importance of school-family collaboration and communication is evident in a community crisis such as this. What suggestions would you give the school-based safety and crisis teams at Simpson Elementary School about how they could have / should have fostered communication with families before and after this storm? (**D7**)

7. If some of the teachers report feeling overwhelmed upon the return to school, is it appropriate for the school to provide support for the adults who work in the building? Why or why not? If yes, what types of support for staff could be recommended? (**O2, O4**)

Advanced Applications

1. Using Table 6.1, create lists that detail specific areas that the crisis team should focus on in both the short-term (acute stage of this crisis) and in the long-term recovery efforts for the school community efforts. (**D6**)

Table 6.1 Crisis Team Planning Document

Day After Storm Response	1st Week After Storm Response	1st Month After Storm Response	2–6 Months After Storm Response	Summer Prior to Reopening of School	1st Month of New School Year

2. Design potential survey questions that could be used to evaluate the crisis response from this school for various stakeholders (parents, students, school staff). Include at least 5 survey questions that could be asked of each stakeholder group. **(D7, D9)**
3. Suppose that by November of the next school year, your Child Study Team is reporting a much higher than usual referral rate for special education evaluation and eligibility due to increased academic concerns of both teachers and parents. How would you handle this situation? What data might you need to collect to better understand what is going on with these children related to their academic progress? **(D3)**
4. Review and summarize the chapter by Heath (2014) *Best Practices in Crisis Intervention Following a Natural Disaster*. Based on these practices, what else should the school consider doing in response to this storm? **(D6)**

Case Two: An Ill-Advised Promise of Confidentiality

Christina is a 15-year-old White sophomore student who the school psychologist, Mr. Davies, has been concerned about for some time. She comes to see the school psychologist and indicates that she has something she needs to talk to him about, but that he must swear to keep it a secret. Mr. Davies is pleased that Christina has come to see him because he has reached out to her several times in the past year due to concerns about drinking and possible drug use reported by teachers; however, she has not been interested in engaging with him. Now she has suddenly come to his office and Mr. Davies feels like it would be best to promise confidentiality to her so that she will open up to him about her concerns. He is quite surprised when she comes into his office and begins to talk about her concerns about her friend, rather than herself. Christina indicates that for the past week, she has been really worried about Jessie, another student at the school. Christina reports that Jessie's girlfriend has recently broken up with him and he has been despondent over the breakup. He was also fired from his job at a retail store due to suspicions by the manager that he had stolen money from the register. He does not know if the manager will be pressing charges against him and he is terrified that his parents will find out about the theft and that he has gotten fired.

Christina has been on the phone with him for the past several nights until three or four a.m. as he cries and tells her that there is no reason to go on living. She has been staying on the phone with him all night because she is concerned that he will harm himself if she gets off the phone with him. She also reported that he has been leaving for work as usual during his scheduled shifts so that his parents do not find out that he has been fired. During his scheduled work times, he tells her he goes to sit by the river and thinks about how to end his life. Christina indicates that she needs this to stay a secret but is reaching out to Mr. Davies for advice on how to help Jessie during their late-night phone calls.

Mr. Davies informs Christina that he is genuinely concerned about Jessie and that he will need to speak with Jessie and his parents and other school officials about this situation. Christina becomes irate with Mr. Davies and begins screaming at him in the office about his broken promises. She then runs out of the office and reportedly leaves school grounds. The security guard reports that he witnessed Christina running into the woods surrounding the school property but could not find her once he went to look for her. Mr. Davies is at a loss about how the situation with Christina turned into this type of crisis. He knows that he also now needs to contact Christina's parents to let them know that the school cannot find her.

Discussion Questions

1.   Quite a few things went wrong with Mr. Davies handling of this situation. What ethical mistakes did Mr. Davies make in this situation? (**D10**)
2.   What are Mr. Davies ethical obligations in this situation? (**D10**)

3. What concerns are the most pressing for Mr. Davies at this point? (**D4, D6**)
4. What steps should Mr. Davies immediately take now to ensure the safety of both students involved? (**D4, D6**)
5. Mr. Davies motives are to establish a relationship with Christina to assist her during counseling. What are some other ways that he could have gone about trying to establish a relationship with her so that he could assist her? (**D4**)
6. Should Mr. Davies be reprimanded for his actions in this case by the principal at the school? By his own supervisor? Why or why not? (**O1**)

Advanced Applications

1. What specific ways should Mr. Davies follow up with Christina and her family that day and also the following day in school? (**D4, D6, D7**)
2. Mr. Davies decides to immediately follow up with Jessie and his family. Research an appropriate suicide risk assessment that could be utilized in this situation. (**D1, D4**)
3. What types of professional development do you recommend for Mr. Davies to assist him in better understanding best practices for future situations such as this one? (**O6**)
4. Review and summarize the *Best Practices in Suicide Prevention and Intervention* chapter (Lieberman et al., 2014). According to the practices set forth in this chapter, what should Mr. Davies have done differently? How should he respond now? (**D4, D6**)

Case Three: Threat Assessment Gone Wrong?

Brendan is an eighth-grade student at the middle school who receives special education services due to a diagnosis of autism. Previous testing has indicated that he has low cognitive abilities. He receives special education services in the self-contained Multiple Disabilities program at the middle school. Recently, his self-contained teacher has reported concerns that Brendan has developed an interest in an eighth-grade girl, Ava, who also attends the school. The teacher fears that he is becoming preoccupied with his interests in Ava. He reportedly has become angry with her when she has not paid attention to him when they see each other in school. He has had some angry outbursts when he feels slighted by Ava, but these outbursts have occurred after he has returned to his self-contained classroom. Thus far, the teacher has been successful in calming him down after a few minutes. The school psychologist, Mrs. Larrimone, has consulted with the teacher about this issue and has begun working with Brendan in their already scheduled counseling sessions about how to communicate more appropriately with his peers and about appropriate reactions when feeling slighted or ignored by others. These sessions appear to be making a difference and Brendan's teacher had just come to the school psychologist to report an improvement in Brendan's interactions and reactions to his peers overall. Mrs. Larrimone has been doing her own research to ensure that she has the skills to discuss the changes associated with puberty with Brendan in appropriate ways. She plans to begin having these discussions with Brendan in the next session.

However, just one day later, the school psychologist finds out that Ava's parents have called the principal to report that Brendan has threatened their daughter. They indicate that she is now extremely afraid to go to lunch because he had said to her "if you don't sit by me, I will get you and all of your friends too." The parents are extremely concerned that this was a threat to their daughter. The principal investigates the situation by speaking with Ava and her friends who all witnessed Brendan make this comment. The principal also speaks with Brendan's self-contained classroom teacher and learns about the ongoing concern regarding Brendan's seeming preoccupation with Ava. Unfortunately, the school psychologist, Mrs. Larrimone, was in a meeting in another building when this all occurs so she is not aware of the situation until the end of the day.

After speaking with the self-contained teacher, the principal attempts to speak to Brendan about the situation. However, since the principal and Brendan do not have a good rapport and have had limited interactions in the past, Brendan does not respond to the principal's questions and he becomes agitated. The principal then makes the decision to call the police to report Brendan's threat. Brendan becomes extremely frightened when the police arrive and ends up acting out in aggressive ways. He backs himself into a corner when the police officer is trying to speak to him and begins crying and screaming. This situation escalates until Brendan throws books from a nearby shelf at the principal and police officer. This unfortunately leads to Brendan's arrest and he leaves the school in handcuffs.

Discussion Questions

1. This situation escalated to the point where the police were called. Review the steps taken by the school and indicate the points in which the school staff could have made different decisions to diffuse this situation. (**D6**)

2. What are the implications of using zero tolerance policies in schools? (**D6**)
3. What are the controversies related to the potential concern of "over-policing" in schools? (**D6**)
4. How should the school balance the needs of Brendan and the safety of Ava? (**D6**)
5. What are the ethical implications of various decisions that were made in this situation? (**D10**)
6. Brendan's parents did not seem to be included in these discussions about the concern from his teacher about the angry outbursts. When should his parents have been brought into the discussion? How might this have changed the outcome? (**D7**)

Advanced Applications

1. Research a threat assessment that might have been productive for use in this situation. Why did you select this assessment (pros/cons)? (**D6**)
2. What are best practices for utilizing School Resource Officers in schools? (**D6**)
3. How might this school's specific climate have contributed to how the situation was eventually handled? How could the school focus on the issues of climate in the future to avoid this type of outcome? (**O2**)
4. Review Cornell (2014) *Best Practices in Threat Assessment in Schools*. Summarize Cornell's major points regarding best practices in threat assessment and apply these practices to this case.

Case Four: Perceptions of Climate

A school-wide climate survey was distributed to all students, teachers and parents in a large middle school that serves children in grades six through eight. The survey asked similar questions to parents, students, and teachers to get their perceptions of bullying and other school climate issues in the school. Table 6.2 provides data regarding the percentage of responses that indicated participant agreement (agree or strongly agree) to the statements provided. The survey included a four-point Likert scale (Strongly Disagree, Disagree, Agree, Strongly Agree). See Table 6.2 and Figure 6.1, which present the results of this school-wide climate survey.

Table 6.2 School Community Responses to School Climate Survey

Climate Survey Question (Student Version/Teacher and Parent Version)	Student Responses	Teacher/Staff Responses	Parent Responses
Bullying is a problem at my school.	89%	35%	71%
I feel safe at school. (Children feel safe at school.)	42%	85%	60%
I feel like I belong at this school. (This school fosters a sense of belonging for children.)	65%	91%	85%
I have reported bullying to a teacher in the past month. (Bullying has been reported to me in the past month.)	28%	4%	35%
When I report bullying to a teacher, something is done about it. (When bullying is reported, we investigate and handle the situation.)	49%	97%	68%
I am comfortable talking to the principal/vice-principal about bullying situations. (Students feel comfortable talking to the principal/vice-principal about bullying situations).	32%	45%	20%
Our school has a specific policy and procedures for reporting bullying, harassment, or assault at school?	45%	95%	82%
In general, my school is a safe school.	60%	91%	74%
In general, my school is a supportive and positive place.	30%	87%	72%

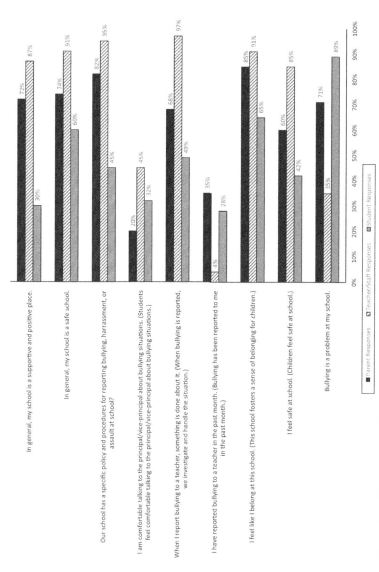

Figure 6.1 Climate Survey Results

The middle school results were like those found by Bradshaw et al. (2007) regarding perception differences amongst children and staff. These items come from their web-based survey adapted from a school climate and aggression survey (Institute of Behavioral Science, 1990), bullying research (Nansel et al., 2001; Solberg & Olweus, 2003) and attitudes towards retaliation from the Normative Beliefs About Aggression Scale (Huesmann et al., 1992). This study found that staff were more likely to report that children feel safe and have a sense of belonging at school than the children reported. Similarly, the students were more likely than the teachers to report the acceptability of the use of aggression/force for retaliation. The school staff was more likely to indicate that bullying was reported to them in the past month (45.6 percent of staff) when compared to the students (21.3 percent). Regarding the staff response to bullying, 33 percent of children reported that nothing was done when they reported bullying to staff, while only 0.6 percent of teachers indicated that they ignore or do nothing when bullying is reported to them.

Discussion Questions

1. According to Bradshaw et al. (2007), this issue is common. What is the school psychologist's role in understanding these differences in perception in their own schools and making decisions about prevention, intervention, and response? (**D6**)

2. For those in field placements, do these data already exist at your field placement site and is anyone analyzing and discussing it? What does that look like? If not, what is the school psychologist's role in working with the school to review, select, and adopt similar screening measures? (**D1**)

3. Staff members' perceived efficacy for resolving a bullying situation is highly related to their likelihood of intervening effectively (Bradshaw et al., 2007; Nicolaides et al., 2002). What is the school psychologist's role in working to increase staff efficacy to handle these issues? (**D2**)

4. According to Bradshaw et al. (2007), teachers may not always respond to a bullying report if there is a perceived lack of administrative support, lack of a school-wide policy regarding bullying, or if the culture of the school does not promote bullying prevention. This can lead to a passive approach to bullying response. What is the role of the school psychologist in working with administration to address these organizational issues? (**D6, O4**)

Advanced Applications

1. Review bullying assessment tools available (e.g., Hamburger et al., 2011). Compare and contrast at least two different measures to identify the advantages and limitations of each.
2. Identify evidence-based resources and programs that this school might use to create a more positive school climate. (**D5, D9**)
3. Create a short presentation to present at a school staff meeting to present this data and solicit feedback about what might be causing these differences in perspective between students and teachers. (**D1, D2, D6, O4**)
4. What ideas might be used to allow parents/families to get more involved in creating a positive school climate? (**D7, O2**)
5. Review the "Best Practices in Bullying Prevention" chapter (Felix et al., 2014). Based on their suggested practices, what else should the school be working on to decrease the problem of bullying within the school? (**D5, D6**)

References

Bradshaw, C. P., Sawyer, A. L., & O'Brennan, L. M. (2007). Bullying and peer victimization at school: Perceptual differences between students and school staff. *School Psychology Review, 36*(3), 361–382. https://doi.org/10.1080/02796015.2007.12087929

Brock, S., Nickerson, A., Louvar Reeves, C., Conolly, J. S., Pesce, R., & Lazzaro, B. (2016). *School crisis prevention and intervention: The PREPaRE model* (2nd ed.). National Association of School Psychologists.

Cornell, D. (2014). Best practices in threat assessment in schools. In P. L. Harrison & A. Thomas (Eds.), *Best practices in school psychology: Systems-level services* (pp. 259–272). National Association of School Psychologists.

Felix, E. D., Green, J. G., & Sharkey, J. D. (2014). Best practices in bullying prevention. In P. L. Harrison & A. Thomas (Eds.), *Best practices in school psychology: Systems-level services* (pp. 245–258). National Association of School Psychologists.

Hamburger, M. E., & Basile, K. C., & Vivolo, A. M. (2011). *Measuring bullying victimization, perpetration, and bystander experiences: A compendium of assessment tools.* Centers for Disease Control and Prevention, National Center for Injury Prevention and Control. https://stacks.cdc.gov/view/cdc/5994

Heath, M. A. (2014). Best practices in crisis intervention following a natural disaster. In P. L. Harrison & A. Thomas (Eds.), *Best practices in school psychology: Systems-level services* (pp. 289–302). National Association of School Psychologists.

Huesmann, R., Guerra, N., Miller, L., & Zelli, A. (1992). The role of social norms in the development of aggression. In H. Zumkley & A. Fraczek (Eds.), *Socialization and aggression.* Springer.

Institute of Behavioral Science. (1990). *Youth interview schedule: Denvery youth survey.* Unpublished manuscript, University of Colorado, Boulder.

Lieberman, R., Poland, S., & Kornfeld, C. (2014). Best practices in suicide prevention and intervention. In P. L. Harrison & A. Thomas (Eds.), *Best practices in school psychology: Systems-level services* (pp. 273–288). National Association of School Psychologists.

Nansel, T. R., Overpeck, M., Pilla, R. S., Ruan, W. J., Simons-Morton, B., & Scheidt, P. (2001). Bullying behaviors among US youth. *Jama, 285*(16), 2094. https://doi.org/10.1001/jama.285.16.2094

National Association of School Psychology. (2020). *The professional standards of the national association of school psychologists.* National Association of School Psychologists.

Nicolaides, S., Toda, Y., & Smith, P. K. (2002). Knowledge and attitudes about school bullying in trainee teachers. *British Journal of Educational Psychology, 72*(1), 105–118. https://doi.org/10.1348/000709902158793

Solberg, M. E., & Olweus, D. (2003). Prevalence estimation of school bullying with the Olweus Bully/Victim Questionnaire. *Aggressive Behavior, 29*(3), 239–268. https://doi.org/10.1002/ab.10047

School Psychologists as Family, School, and Community Collaborators

7

Domain 7: Family, School, and Community Collaboration

"School psychologists understand principles and research related to family systems, strengths, needs, and cultures; evidence-based strategies to support positive family influences on children's learning and mental health; and strategies to develop collaboration between families and schools. School psychologists, in collaboration with others, design, implement, and evaluate services that respond to culture and context. They facilitate family and school partnerships and interactions with community agencies to enhance academic and social-behavioral outcomes for children." (NASP, 2020, p. 8)

The importance of positive family-school relationships on the positive development of children has been well documented in the literature. For example, in their meta-analysis of the impact of family-school relationships on children's social-emotional development and mental health, Sheridan et al. (2019) found significant positive effects of family-school interventions on children's social-emotional development. NASP has also created a position statement highlighting the importance of positive school-family partnerships that includes the important elements for success in creating and maintaining these successful partnerships (NASP, 2019). When working collaboratively with families to understand and solve issues and concerns, school psychologists and schools, in general, can have a greater chance of success. To develop positive and collaborative relationships with families, school psychologists must understand the diversity within and across families in the communities where work, including various communication styles and family expectations of schools. School psychologists must have the ability to understand that their own worldviews and biases must not affect how they interact and develop relationships with families with differing worldviews.

The establishment of inclusive and welcoming school communities are critical for the development of trust and positive relationships between schools and the families they serve. School psychologists should collaborate with other school personnel to ensure that policies and practices are inclusive of the families within their school community. This may happen by creating school-community events, ensuring that meetings and events are scheduled at times that can work for most of the families within the school, or creating an atmosphere of inclusiveness for families by inviting parents to take part in class and school-wide events. School psychologists should strive to ensure that parents and other caregivers feel like their voices are important in advocating for the needs of their children. Parents should understand that their input as the expert on their own child is valued by school personnel. To this end, school psychologists should ensure that staff understand the vast benefits of creating positive school-family partnerships and how these partnerships can allow for proper supports and interventions for children. The first case focuses on the critical need for foster parents to feel heard in an IEP meeting. When parents leave a meeting frustrated and feeling "unheard" or when the team misses an opportunity to understand the valuable input of the parent, the school is not likely to be able to effectively support to the child. Discussion questions focus on how the school team might have handled this specific IEP meeting better. The fourth case highlights the critical need for parents to understand the special education eligibility process and how school psychologists should work to ensure that assessment results are understandable and relatable to their primary readers, the parents of the child being evaluated.

School psychologists must actively work to support minoritized students and their families within the school environment. This may include collaborating and developing relationships with community providers to provide necessary support for these children. When children are involved with multiple community agencies, school psychologists can serve as the link between these community groups and the school environment to ensure that consistent messaging and idea sharing (with permission) is used. Community-wide partnerships may be set up to create continuity of care and ensure the education of all direct service providers for a child and family. Both the second and third cases focus on how schools can effectively partner with community agencies to provide students and families with necessary supports. This includes a community agency that provides bilingual services and a community agency that educates the school on visually impaired services, respectively.

The four cases within this chapter all highlight the vital importance of forging effective family, school, and community partnerships to ensure student success. The cases vary from demonstrating problematic interactions that hinder successful partnerships to more effective best practices in how to develop positive relationships with our vital partners in education. In all four cases, there are many opportunities to reflect upon how to improve practices to ensure more positive and effective relationships with families and communities.

Case One: Fostering Relationships

Jamal, a fifth-grade Black student, had entered foster care with his sibling at age 18-months due to ongoing neglect issues. He lived with his foster family for about one and a half years and then was reunified with his biological family. Due to more neglect and suspected physical abuse, Jamal was again removed from his biological family's home again at the end of first grade and placed with the same foster family who he had originally been placed with as a toddler. His foster family was white and recently moved out of the city to the suburbs for a house that could accommodate Jamal and his sibling along with their other biological children. At the start of second grade, Jamal enrolled in a new school where his foster family lived. This meant that Jamal moved from a predominantly Black urban school to a predominantly White suburban school. Once he started at the new school, there was no new student welcome or support group counseling sessions offered by the school. He seemed to adjust well to the transition despite the absence of those types of resources. Even with his background of trauma and the recent upheaval and transitions in his life, he appeared happy and made friends easily.

After a few months of school, Jamal started having trouble in school. His teachers contacted his foster parent, Ms. Kramer, to discuss concerns often. They reported that he would have a tantrum, pout, bang his desk, and refuse to do his work, creating such a distraction that the behavior spe-cialist would remove him from class temporarily to cool down. His math teacher specifically was frustrated with Jamal's behavior in her class and felt he would do better in the other second grade math teacher's class, which was also on grade level, but "a little less challenging." Ms. Kramer was not thrilled about this plan. She was concerned that Jamal was being placed in a lower-level math group. She wanted to focus more on the development of interventions and not just move Jamal to another classroom. At the same time, she realized it might not help to push for Jamal to stay in a teacher's classroom who was not willing to make changes to her instructional or behavioral approach. Ms. Kramer agreed to the switch of math classes, but asked for a team meeting to talk about an intervention with the school's Student Support Team (SST).

At the first SST meeting, the new second grade math teacher, Mr. Ful-ton, said that he felt Jamal's math accuracy and limited math fact fluency was due to his difficulty paying attention. The teacher suggested that they try to implement a new intervention. He suggested that they allow Jamal to chew gum to increase his focus in class. Ms. Kramer, a former teacher, knew that was not going to be an effective intervention. She was frustrated with this "chewing gum intervention" but tried to stay posi-tive in the meeting with the goal of keeping good school relationships. Ms. Kramer did try to say that chewing gum was not a research-based intervention. She agreed that Jamal would enjoy chewing gum, but that it would not help increase his ability to focus or increase his math skills. Mr. Fulton said that chewing gum is what helped him as a child, so Ms. Kramer did not argue and agreed that they could try it for now. She did state that she believed that his tantrums in math were due to difficulty in math, not due to lack of focus. She could see at home during his home-work that he worked well and focused when he was working on addition facts, but that he would whine and complain when he received subtrac-tion problems. She felt that it was important to note that working on math skills might help his focus and reduce his tantrums, as opposed to the other way around. She asked that other interventions be considered beyond the chewing gum.

After the SST meeting, Ms. Kramer received the minutes of the meet-ing in the mail. After reading the minutes, she was concerned that her comments about the math difficulty were not well documented in the notes, nor were her requests for a math intervention. She noticed that the teacher's comments about the potential cause of the difficulty were well documented. The report read, "Jamal's lack of math accuracy and fluency is due to his difficulty focusing." Ms. Kramer requested revisions to the minutes. She either wanted the causal statement to be removed completely or at least be revised to qualify it by saying, "Mr. Fulton *believes* the math accuracy and fluency is due to lack of focus." She also asked for an addition of the alternate viewpoint, "Ms. Kramer believes the lack of focus could be due to difficulty accurately and fluently solving math problems." The school SST Chair refused to revise the minutes. Ms. Kramer asserted that math fluency and accuracy errors may lead to lack of focus and that causation could not be proven from the assessments that were conducted. She explained that a more specific definition of the problem is important to deciding interventions. The IEP Chair suggested that Ms. Kramer meet with the principal to discuss her concerns. Once she met with the principal, Ms. Kramer was even more frustrated that the principal disagreed with her request. The principal said that Ms. Kramer could write an addendum to appeal. Ms. Kramer disagreed because she did not feel that she was trying to change the facts of the meeting. She felt that the minutes just did not accurately portray what was said at the meeting. The principal stayed firm in her decision not to revise the minutes. Ms. Kramer left the meeting with the principal feeling angry and hopeless that this school was able to help Jamal.

Discussion Questions

1. How did communication in the meetings or after the meetings affect parent and school relationships? (**D7**)
2. Assuming the school psychologist was at this meeting, what could they have done differently to maintain relationships? (**D7, D10**)
3. What is the school psychologist's role in consulting with the teachers before or after the meeting? If you were the school psychologist, how would you have followed-up with the teachers or staff after each meeting? (**D2, D3, D4, D7, D10**)
4. How is the school helping to close the gap for students with a significant background of trauma or for students of color? What barriers might they be putting in place for the family? (**D7, D8**)
5. What other supports might be needed for this family in addition to academic problem-solving? (**D3, D7**)
6. What are the parents' rights to request meeting minutes be redacted or revised? When should we make requested revisions versus when should a parent addendum be added? (**D7, D10**)

Advanced Applications

1. What could the school have done to try to identify if the math accuracy and fluency issue were due to attentional difficulties or math skills? What assessments would you recommend? **(D1, D3, D4)**

2. Review the research on gum-chewing and on-task behavior? Is there any evidence to support that practice? What evidence-based interventions would be better to suggest besides gum chewing? **(D3, D4, D9)**

3. In the scenario, there was no plan to monitor the progress of the gum chewing intervention after the SST meeting. What assessments would you suggest for progress-monitoring? **(D1)**

4. Review the Kendrick-Dunn et al. (2020) article *Infusing Social Justice into Tiered Service Delivery for Low-Income and Economically Marginalized Students in Foster Care* and discuss recommendations for this case based on the reading. **(D7, D8, D10)**

5. Review Scherr (2014) chapter "Best Practices in Working With Children Living in Foster Care" and discuss recommendations for this case based on the best practices discussed in the chapter. **(D7, D8, D10)**

6. Is an FBA warranted in this case? Why or why not?

7. If you were to recommend that an FBA be completed, what steps would you take to complete this FBA? Review the chapter by Steege and Scheib (2014) entitled "Best Practices in Conducting Functional Behavioral Assessments" to assist in your response.

Case Two: Language Differences or Deficits?

As a new school psychologist at Elm Tree Elementary, Ms. Lupita started noticing some cultural clashes between the school staff and families. The school consisted of 35 percent Hispanic/Latinx students, 49 percent Black students, 14 percent White students, and 2 percent students identifying with more than two races. Additionally, 65 percent of the students in the school qualify for free/reduced lunch, indicating that they come from economically disadvantaged backgrounds. Speaking to the Community Resource Coordinator of the school, Mrs. Hernandez, Ms. Lupita quickly learned that there had been a recent influx of families from Guatemala and El Salvador. Mrs. Hernandez said that most of the teachers in the school, who are primarily white females, assume that the students are all from Mexico. She said that the teachers often do not take the time to learn more about their students' cultural heritage. Mrs. Hernandez also noted that, in general, the staff in the school have a low opinion of the students' families because they do not attend parent conferences or meetings to a high degree. In terms of student achievement, 58 percent of the English learners (ELs) in the school are making progress on the annual state assessment, however only 11 percent are at or above proficient in math and language arts. Alternatively, 75 percent of the white students in the school are at or above proficient.

One day, Ms. Lupita came to school and noticed a mother attempting to use the automated school check-in system while bringing her children to school late. Because the system is entirely in English with no options for alternate languages, the parent was having a lot of difficulty and had to have her children help her to translate. Before Ms. Lupita could help, the receptionist came over to help the parent, but the receptionist seemed annoyed that the mother did not understand how to use the system. On a different occasion, Ms. Lupita noticed that the school website is entirely in English and translated forms and documents such as the school handbook are either not available or are difficult to find on the website. At a few meetings, Ms. Lupita noticed that translators were not typically present to help translate and interpret for parents who did not speak English. The team members often spoke louder or slower to try to help parents understand. At one meeting, a parent requested a translator and when one was not available, she asked for the meeting to be rescheduled for when a translator would be available. The teacher seemed exasperated after the meeting that they would now have to reschedule for another day.

While this was upsetting for Ms. Lupita to see the many ways linguistically different families were experiencing frustrations and barriers, she was pleased to see some of the improvements the school was making. For example, the school recently hired Mrs. Hernandez as the Community Resource Coordinator. In this new role, Mrs. Hernandez established a family resource room for bilingual parents. She started to hold workshops with translation. The parent attendance at those sessions was high. She started to translate at the PTA meetings and provided families with a headset to hear the translated version of the meetings. Attendance at those meetings was also starting to increase.

Discussion Questions

1. What is the school psychologists' role to support the Community Resource Coordinator in supporting the linguistically diverse families of this school? (**D7, D8, D10**)

2. What teacher supports and services are needed? (**D2, D7, D8**)
3. In what ways might the school staff need to develop their own multi-cultural competency? Review the chapter from Miranda (2014) entitled "Best Practices in Increasing Cross-Cultural Competency" and discuss the ideas listed within the chapter about how to begin the process of increasing cross-cultural competency. (**D8, D10, O6**)
4. What are the ethical and/or legal issues present in this case? What is the school psychologists' role in addressing these issues? (**D8, D10**)
5. What academic equity issues are evident in this case? (**D1, D3, D8**)

Advanced Applications

1. What assessment steps might you recommend to better understand the academic equity issues at this school? (**D1, D3, D8**)
2. Research evidence-based practices for working with linguistically diverse families for improving academic outcomes for students. (**D2, D3, D7, D8, D9**)
3. Develop a list of recommendations and guidelines for working with translators and interpreters in your school, based on best practices. (**D7, D10**)
4. Review the chapter by Vanderwood and Socie (2014) entitled "Best Practices in Assessing and Improving English Language Learners' Literacy Performance." Based on their recommendations, what factors would you suggest that this school needs to be considered to improve academic scores for all children?
5. Review "Best Practices in Working With Children From Economically Disadvantaged Backgrounds" (Mulé et al., 2014). According to these authors, what are some of the risk and protective factors that should be considered when working with children from economically disadvantaged backgrounds? How can these risk and protective factors be applied in this case to ensure school-wide processes that support these children? (**D5, D6, D7**)

Case Three: Expanding the School's Knowledge Base: Collaborating With Family and Community Agencies

Daphne is an incoming White, kindergarten student in a midsize suburban school district. Her family recently moved to the area from a neighboring state. Daphne is legally blind and received special education services for her visual impairment through her previous pre-school since birth. The school psychologist, Mr. Jackson, and the rest of the IEP team at her new kindergarten have not worked with a student who is legally blind. Initially, they were concerned that they lacked the knowledge to create an effective program for the student. Given this situation, the school psychologist and team first consulted with the parents of the student when they became aware Daphne was entering the district. Daphne's mother attended two team meetings over the summer to provide information about her daughter (strengths and weaknesses) and provide information about her daughter's specific needs within the school building, effective classroom design and physical setup of space. She also shared the academic, social, and emotional needs of her daughter, specifically, as well as the needs of children who are blind in general.

The team learned a lot from the parent about the needs of both her daughter, and the blind community in general, and they valued her expertise. The parent also expressed how appreciative she was that the team was so open to collaborating and communicating with her about her daughter. Next, the team reached out to the Commission for the Blind and Visually Impaired in their state to learn more. From that communication, the commission put them in touch with a local community agency that aids schools in professional development for visually impaired youth. The kindergarten teacher, the administrative team, and members of the Child Study Team all attended training by this community agency over the summer. Finally, with a representative from the Commission for the Blind and Visually Impaired, they scheduled Orientation and Mobility sessions with Daphne and her family prior to the beginning of the school year. The commission also assisted the district in understanding the various instructional technology and supports that Daphne needed to progress academically with her peers. The school reviewed resources about the expanded curriculum that will be specific to this child, which included specific vision-related skills written into Daphne's IEP (i.e., learning how to use various technologies, learning Braille, learning how to use the vision that she does have efficiently). In consultation with all the various experts, it was decided that Daphne will learn Braille in school, while continuing to focus on key academic skills, such as focusing on phonemic awareness skills to aid the development of reading skills.

While Daphne's mother was anxious about her daughter starting kindergarten, particularly in a new community and school, she felt that the district was responsive and open to her family's concerns and needs. Even before school started, there were open lines of communication between the school and parents, as well as the school and the local community agencies with expertise in supporting visually impaired children. This leads to a positive rapport and feelings of trust between the family and the school. Daphne's mother indicated that she was particularly pleased to see how the various professionals at the school were so open to learning from the various community experts. When the school year began in September, the school and family were prepared to provide Daphne with a positive educational experience. The kindergarten teacher indicated that she was in touch via email with the community agency who offered her ongoing support in designing her instructional plan. Together with the well-trained paraprofessional in the classroom, the school year started for Daphne in a successful manner.

Discussion Questions

1. The school initially was concerned that they may not have the necessary expertise to support a child moving into their district with a visual impairment. What specific steps did they take to ensure that they learned what was necessary to create a sound plan for Daphne's education? (**D7**)

2. The case shows the value of effective collaborations with families as well as community agencies. What was the positive outcome of these collaborations? What if the team had not been as proactive in reaching out to the family and community agencies with the expertise needed? What could have been the result? (**D7**)

3. What types of ongoing collaboration with outside agencies would you suggest to ensure that the team continues to understand and respond to Daphne's needs? What types of ongoing professional development would you suggest? (**D8, D10, O6**)

4. In this case, the parent becomes the consultant to the school, in that she provides them with necessary information both about her daughter and about the potential needs in general of students with visual impairments. The school is receptive to receiving this information from Daphne's mother. This leads to a collaborative consultation between the school and family that can have ongoing benefits as Daphne progresses in school. How might the mother's role as expert assist the collaborative relationship in the future? (**D2**)

5. Contrast how the school collaborates with Daphne's mother with how the school collaborates with Jamal's mother in Case One. How does the school value the parent's expertise differently in these two cases? (**D7**)

Advanced Applications

1. Research the available resources in your community for students with visual impairments. Create a list of community supports/agencies that are available to potentially provide support to schools. (**D7**)
2. Research available resources for at least two other low-incidence disabilities and create a list of these resources. (**D7**)
3. Conduct a literature review about best practices for supporting children in schools with low-incidence disabilities. Summarize best practices for school-based teams. (**D7**)
4. While all children with visual impairments will have different strengths/needs as well as differing levels of support needed to progress academically in schools, research some common technologies and services that may be used in schools for children with visual impairments. (**D8**)
5. According to Bradley-Johnson and Cook (2014) in their "Best Practices in School-Based Services for Students With Visual Impairments" chapter, schools must be aware of and respond to various potential needs of visually impaired children in several areas, including academic development, social skills, classroom behavior, and physical activity/exercise. Research some potential challenges for children with visually impaired students in each of these stated areas and include best practice approaches for how schools should provide accommodations and interventions for these students. (**D3, D4**)

Case Four: Who Is This Report Written for Anyway?

Kenny is a White, second-grade student who was referred for an evaluation by both his teacher and mother due to ongoing concerns with his academic performance, as well as behavioral concerns in the classroom. His mother had first requested a school meeting last year when he was in first grade because she was concerned that he was falling behind in reading. She was often called by Kenny's teacher about his behavioral outbursts. She was worried that he was frustrated because he was struggling with reading. At the time, the Child Study Team (CST) decided not to proceed forward with an evaluation because they felt he seemed immature for his age and that he would likely "catch-up" by second or third grade. Now in second grade, his behavioral outbursts and poor academic performance have continued, and his teacher has also asked that he be evaluated. This year, the Child Study Team agrees that Kenny should be evaluated to decide if he needs special education services.

Kenny's mom, Ms. Linus, received several reports prior to the scheduled meeting with the school. She read all the reports thoroughly but has many questions about what the different tests and numbers mean. She found the narrative of the report to be so jargon-filled that she had trouble following what was being said. She called the school and when connected to the CST Secretary, Ms. Linus asked whether there was a glossary of terms available so that she could understand the terminology. The secretary told her that there was no such glossary available but assured her that while the reports are difficult to understand, the team of professionals would explain it all to her in the meeting. Therefore, Ms. Linus looked forward to the discussion with the school.

When she attended the meeting, she was dismayed that there was no opportunity for discussion. The same professionals who created the reports took turns reading the report in the meeting, used the same jargon and simply reported scores that were presented in the report. After each professional finished reading their reports, the team indicated that he qualified as a student with a learning disability and asked the mom if she agreed. She did not have time to ask her questions and she was not sure why they decided he qualified for services. Based on her experience from first grade, she believed that the only avenue for her son to receive reading help was through qualification for special education services, so she agreed that he qualified. However, she did not actually know what guidelines they were using to say he qualified. She was about to take out her list of questions about the reports that she had prepared in advance, when the secretary came into the meeting to say that the next parent had arrived for their scheduled meeting. The team told the parent that if she had any other questions, she could call and talk to the case manager assigned to her child. She was given the case manager's contact information and escorted out of the meeting.

Discussion Questions

1. The title of this case is "Who Is This Report Written For?" Why do you think the case has this title? In your opinion, who should reports be written for? (**D7**)

2. There are several areas of concern related to the way that this process unfolds in this situation. What are the areas of concern? Why are these concerns? Are there any ethical concerns? (**D7, D10**)

3. In what specific ways, could the school team make changes to ensure more effective school-family collaboration? (**D7**)
4. School teams may often indicate that the reports will be explained at the meeting to discuss findings. What are the barriers to doing this effectively? What sort of procedural changes in schools might be necessary to ensure that meetings are more parent-friendly? (**D7, O3, O2**)
5. In what specific ways can school-based teams reflect on how they present results to parents in meetings? What are specific ways to make changes to evaluation findings meetings to make them more parent- and child-focused? (**D7, O3**)
6. In all stages of this evaluation process, this case highlights ways in which Ms. Linus attempted to collaborate with the school regarding her concerns about her son's academic and behavioral performance. List the ways in which she tried to collaborate and the results of those efforts. (**D7**)

Advanced Applications

1. Review some of the research on report-writing, including *Best Practices in Writing Assessment Reports* (Walrath et al., 2014). What are the major findings related to best practices in presenting results to parents? (**D7**)
2. Integrated, theme-based, or referral-based reports may be more easily understood as well as more practical for parents/teachers and may more easily lend themselves to recommendations. Find examples of one or more of these types of reports and analyze the differences between this style of report and a more typical test-by-test presentation of findings. (**D1, D7**)
3. Role play an efficient way to present assessment results in meetings that are brief yet leave time for collaborative conversations between school professional and parents. (**D7**)
4. Review some of the best practices presented in Minke and Jensen's chapter *"Best Practices in Facilitating Family-School Meetings"* (2014). What strategies presented in this chapter could have applied in this case? (**D7**)
5. When concerns about Kenny's performance first arose in first grade, the school indicated that he would likely "catch-up" and that he was just immature for his age. Discuss the major problems with this type of approach to children who are beginning to fall behind academically in first grade. (**D3**)

References

Bradley-Johnson, S., & Cook, A. (2014). Best practices in school-based services for students with visual impairments. In P. L. Harrison & A. Thomas (Eds.), *Best practices in school psychology: Foundations* (pp. 243–254). National Association of School Psychologists.

Kendrick-Dunn, T. B., Barrett, C., Guttman-Lapin, D., Shriberg, D., Proctor, S. L., & Calderón, O. (2020). Infusing social justice into tiered service delivery for low-income and economically marginalized students in foster care. *Communiqué, 48*(6), 1, 22–26.

Minke, K. M., & Jensen, K. L. (2014). Best practices in facilitating family-school meetings. In P. L. Harrison & A. Thomas (Eds.), *Best practices in school psychology: Systems-level services* (pp. 505–518). National Association of School Psychologists.

Miranda, A. H. (2014). Best practices in increasing cross-cultural competency. In P. L. Harrison & A. Thomas (Eds.), *Best practices in school psychology: Foundations* (pp. 9–19). National Association of School Psychologists.

Mulé, C., Briggs, A., & Song, S. (2014). Best practices in working with children from economically disadvantaged backgrounds. In P. L. Harrison & A. Thomas (Eds.), *Best practices in school psychology: Foundations* (pp. 129–142). National Association of School Psychologists.

National Association of School Psychologists. (2019). *School-family partnering to enhance learning: Essential elements and responsibilities* [Position Statement]. National Association of School Psychologists.

National Association of School Psychologists. (2020). *The professional standards of the national association of school psychologists.* National Association of School Psychologists.

Sheridan, S. M., Smith, T. E., Moorman Kim, E., Beretvas, S. N., & Park, S. (2019). A meta-analysis of family-school interventions and children's social-emotional functioning: Moderators and components of efficacy. *Review of Educational Research, 89*(2), 296–332. https://doi.org/10.3102/0034654318825437

Scherr, T. G. (2014). Best practices in working with children living in foster care. In P. L. Harrison & A. Thomas (Eds.), *Best practices in school psychology: Foundations* (pp. 169–180). National Association of School Psychologists.

Steege, M. W., & Scheib, M. A. (2014). Best practices in conducting functional behavioral assessments. In P. L. Harrison & A. Thomas (Eds.), *Best practices in school psychology: Data-based and collaborative decision making* (pp. 273–286). National Association of School Psychologists.

Vanderwood, M. L., & Socie, D. (2014). Best practices in assessing and improving English language learners' literacy performance. In P. L. Harrison & A. Thomas (Eds.), *Best practices in school psychology: Foundations* (pp. 89–98). National Association of School Psychologists.

Walrath, R., Willis, J. O., & Dumont, R. (2014). Best practices in writing assessment reports. In P. L. Harrison & A. Thomas (Eds.), *Best practices in school psychology: Data-based and collaborative decision making* (6th ed., pp. 433–445). National Association of School Psychologists.

Ensuring Equitable Practices for Diverse Populations

8

Domain 8: Equitable Practices for Diverse Populations

"School psychologists have knowledge of individual differences, abilities, disabilities, and other diverse characteristics and the impact they have on development and learning. They also understand principles and research related to diversity in children, families, schools, and communities, including factors related to child development, religion, culture and cultural identity, race, sexual orientation, gender identity and expression, socioeconomic status, and other variables. School psychologists implement evidence-based strategies to enhance services in both general and special education and address potential influences related to diversity. School psychologists demonstrate skills to provide professional services that promote effective functioning for individuals, families, and schools with diverse characteristics, cultures, and backgrounds through an ecological lens across multiple contexts. School psychologists recognize that equitable practices for diverse student populations, respect for diversity in development and learning, and advocacy for social justice are foundational to effective service delivery. While equality ensures that all children have the same access to general and special educational opportunities, equity ensures that each student receives what they need to benefit from these opportunities." (NASP, 2020, p. 8)

As guided by professional ethical principles of fairness, justice, and respect for person's rights and dignity (e.g. NASP, 2020; APA, 2017b), school psychologists must strive to promote equity and respect diversity in all that they do. According to the APA *Multicultural Guidelines* (2017a), psychologists must engage in continual self-reflection to counter their own biases and judgments made about others that might negatively impact diverse children and their families. They also must be aware of how the biases of others influence interactions and the important decisions that are made about children and their families. Whether due to race, gender, sexual orientation, class or any other perceived difference, school psychologists must be aware of and disrupt the biases that negatively affect decisions.

NASP's strategic goal of social justice is to "ensure that all children and youth are valued and that their rights and opportunities are protected in schools and communities" (NASP, 2017). Hence, school psychologists' decisions about how to intervene to support children should be made through a social justice lens. School psychologists should not only embrace social justice, but should move beyond to social justice advocacy, recognizing and proactively addressing injustices, not accepting status quo (Grapin & Kranzler, 2018). Case Two, "Zero Tolerance," highlights the need for social justice advocacy. This case provides an opportunity for discussion about the need for professionals within the school building to understand the student, their culture, their community, and the potential pressures they face navigating their school and community safely. School psychologists are guided by the ethical standard "to correct school practices that are unjustly discriminatory or that deny students or others their legal rights. School psychologists take steps to foster a school climate that is supportive, inclusive, safe, accepting, and respectful toward all persons, particularly those who have experienced marginalization in educational settings" (NASP PPE, 2020, p. 44). Readers should ponder if this standard was upheld fully in this case, as well as what social justice advocacy was needed?

School psychologists must also collaborate with the other professionals within the school and the community to ensure that the community promotes respect for diversity and allows for a supportive school community where all children and their families feel like their voices can be heard. This includes the recognition that children must be understood as the unique individuals that they are, while simultaneously understanding between-group differences. Case Four, "Transition," focuses on a transgender teen's transition to high school, which calls for reflection upon our role with the APA multicultural guideline eight, "Psychologists seek awareness and understanding of how developmental stages and life transitions intersect with the larger biosociocultural context, how identity evolves as a function of such intersections, and how these different socialization and maturation experiences influence worldview and identity" (APA, 2017a, p. 5).

School psychologists should utilize their advanced skills in data analysis to assist in understanding the trends in data that may be negatively impacting diverse students and strive to identify any factors that may be influencing outcomes for diverse children in their academic, social, behavioral, and emotional development. This might include analyzing school-wide discipline data or special education referral rates to determine whether specific groups of students are more at risk for punitive measures or placement in specific types of programming within the school. This data should also be presented to school-based teams and school administrators to remedy issues.

Cases One and Three provide opportunities for discussion related to data-driven decision-making. Specifically, in Case One, "Digging into Discipline Data," the case follows a school psychologist who reveals concerns about equity in school discipline for Black students. The case includes questions that prompt readers to analyze the data and suggest school-wide practices that might contribute to data trends. In Case Three, "Unacclaimed and Underrepresented," readers will discuss a case involving possible inequities in gifted programs. Readers may identify the barriers to equity within the gifted identification procedures and discuss best practices to ensure equity of Black, Latinx, and economically marginalized students. Both cases connect to school psychologists' ethical obligation to correct discrimination and "strive to ensure that all children and youth have equal opportunity to participate in and benefit from school programs and that all students and families have access to and can benefit from school psychological services" (NASP PPE, 2020, p. 44). These cases call for reflection upon the APA's multicultural guideline five, which claims that psychologists are responsible for addressing institutional barriers and inequities (APA, 2017a).

Case One: Digging Into Discipline Data

The school psychologist of a diverse suburban school, Mr. Shields, is an active member of his school's Positive Behavior Intervention Supports (PBIS) Team. Each month, the team reviews their office discipline referral (ODR) data from the SWIS (School-wide Information system). Information about the SWIS processes can be found at www.pbisapps.org/Applications/Pages/SWIS-Suite.aspx. Mr. Shields, along with other team members, usually identify "hot spots," or locations within the school where referrals are the most frequent (e.g., hallway, cafeteria) to analyze the problem and generate solutions. They also look for the 'frequent flyers' to see which students are receiving the most ODRs to determine if more problem-solving is needed. Those students are then referred to the school's Student Support Team (SST) to develop a more targeted or intensive intervention plan. Mr. Shields noticed after a few months of identifying students with frequent referrals that the students who were getting referred to SST were most often Black. He requested that the PBIS Team analyze the ODR data by race and ethnicity at the next meeting. They reviewed the overall demographics for the school in terms of race and ethnicity (see Table 8.1) and then compared that to the data of the percent of students in each racial or ethnic group that received office referrals (see Table 8.2), over the past three years. Mr. Shields was concerned after

Table 8.1 School Demographics: Percentage of Total Enrolled Students

Percent of Enrolled Students			
	2016–2017	2017–2018	2018–2019
Black	36%	33%	36%
Hispanic	8%	11%	12%
White	46%	48%	41%
Other	10%	8%	11%

Table 8.2 School Office Discipline Referrals by Race and Ethnicity: Percentage of the Total Referrals

Percent of Enrolled Students			
	2016–2017	2017–2018	2018–2019
Black	63%	61%	61%
Hispanic	5%	9%	6%
White	28%	28%	31%
Other	4%	2%	1%

reviewing the data and wanted to bring this up to the PBIS Team to see if they could make changes to the discipline procedures to reduce the number of cases coming to the SST. He presented the data in table format to the team and sought their input into what system-level issues might be at work to create this inequitable situation. Unfortunately, the team had difficulty reaching a consensus about the root causes of the problem, with some team members believing that those children just behave in ways that more often justify office referrals. Mr. Shields is concerned that there may be some implicit biases of his fellow team members that are contributing to their viewpoints.

Discussion Questions

1. After reviewing the data, what issues do you see regarding equity for diverse populations? (**D1, D8**)
2. Why is data-based decision-making like this critical to equity for diverse populations in this example? (**D1, D8**)
3. What other data would you want to collect given what you see here? (**D1**)
4. What might you do as a school psychologist in a school that doesn't have a data system like this already in place? (**D2, D3, D4, D5, D6, D7, D8, D9**)
5. How is Mr. Shields' involvement as an active member of this PBIS important for equity for diverse populations? (**D2, D8, O2**)
6. Regarding collaboration and consultation, what should Mr. Shields next steps entail? What process skills should Mr. Shields use? (**D2**)
7. What interventions or next steps should be considered to address this problem school-wide? (**D5, D6**)

Advanced Applications

1. If you are in a field-placement now, ask to review this type of data for your school. Does the school have this type of data readily available? Do they regularly meet to analyze this data, develop action plans, and share the data with staff? Discuss why or why not and the related implications. (**D1, D2**)
2. Research evidence-based practices for school-wide interventions to reduce disproportionate office referrals. (**D5, D6**)
3. Role-play a team meeting where you review the data, assign roles such as school psychologist, teachers, administrator. (**D1, D2**)

4. Create a presentation of this data, including its implications, to include a professional development session for teachers (and administrators). Consider how to best utilize this data for full faculty and/or staff discussions. (**D5, D8**)

Case Two: Zero Tolerance

Ramon, a Latino eighth-grade student, who received special education services for an "other health impairment" due to attentional concerns, attended Rosa Parks Middle School. This school is an urban school with 33 percent White students, 33 percent Black students, and 33 percent Latinx students. The school staff at Rosa Parks were 77 percent White, 13 percent Black, and 10 percent Asian. Ramon lived with his mother and younger siblings. His father was incarcerated. Because Ramon was identified as a student at-risk on a behavior screening survey, he met weekly with his school psychologist, Ms. Hartley, in a small group social-skills intervention with the other students who scored similarly on the universal screening. In group counseling sessions, Ramon was often lethargic or appeared uninterested. The student was also disconnected in his classes, often appeared disengaged, head down in class or playing games on his phone during class. However, he was popular and well liked among his peers. Ms. Hartley was concerned about him. In addition to his group sessions, she occasionally met with him individually to try to establish stronger rapport and find ways to re-engage him.

After several individual and group meetings with Ms. Hartley, Ramon disclosed that he was experimenting with drugs, specifically marijuana. He brought it up in an individual session because he wanted to know what the harmful effects were, if any. As the school psychologist worked with him in a non-judgmental way to research the effects together online, Ramon began to trust her enough to also disclose additional information. At the next session, he told her that he was being recruited to join MS-13. He shared with her that murdering someone was part of the initiation and reported to her his intense fear of getting involved in this type of criminal activity. Despite his moral opposition, he was ambivalent because he also felt he had no escape. He did not feel he could safely turn down the advances of the MS-13 gang members who were approaching him to initiate him. He also worried that he could not report this safely to anyone else or else he could be at great risk.

Ms. Hartley was unsure how to process this heavy information. She had no experience working with students that disclosed gang involvement to her. She empathized with the difficult situation he was in and wanted to do anything to keep him from taking a path that could lead to further harm to himself or others. She tried exploring alternatives with him to see if there would be ways for him to avoid being approached by the gang members. Ramon said he preferred to spend time after school with his uncle in his body shop, but his uncle lived too far for him to walk there, and he couldn't get there consistently or easily. Ms. Hartley tried to encourage the school to look for ways to engage Ramon in after school or community activities to keep him safe after school and away from the gang initiation attempts. Unfortunately, there were not many activities available for him to join easily. As a White female, she was also feeling at a loss for how to connect with him on a deeper level. She urged the school to help find him a Latino mentor. She tried to seek one out for him as well. Her school staff had several male teachers, but none of them were Latino. She then began exploring community resources in the hopes of finding him a mentor or a community group that would also serve as a safe haven for him.

A few weeks later, Ramon was found to have a knife tucked in his sock at school and received a suspension for the offense. Around the same time, the principal reported signs of Ramon's gang involvement to the school district's police and gang task force. Unfortunately, Ramon was found with a knife in his sock another time soon after. He was expelled based on the school's code of conduct for a repeat weapon offense. Ms. Hartley was upset to learn about this decision. She felt strongly that Ramon had no intent to harm anyone and was only carrying the weapon for self-defense. She was worried about what could happen to him, if he did not remain in school and had more time to spend in the community unsupervised. A month later, Ms. Hartley saw Ramon outside of the school on the sidewalk on school grounds, during the school day, wearing a bandana on his face, which she feared was an additional sign of his gang involvement. Not long after that, she saw him on a missing person report on the local news. To her relief, he was eventually found. He never returned to school. She often thought about Ramon and wondered what she or the school could have done differently to help him.

Discussion Questions

1. Discuss the potential socio-cultural mismatches evident in this case and how they may have affected the outcomes. (**D8**)
2. What are some of the ways that the school and community system failed Ramon? What should the individuals involved have done differently to advocate for Ramon? (**D8**)

3. What are your own reactions to this case? How competent do you feel to handle a similar situation? What training or supports would you need, if any? (**D10, O5**)
4. What was Ms. Hartley's level of competence? How did this impact on the decisions that were made? (**D10**)
5. What ethical dilemmas does this case pose? (**D10**)
6. Did Ms. Hartley have a responsibility to intervene immediately once Ramon provided her with information that suggested there was a potential for harm to others? What should she have done at that point? (**D10**)
7. Did Ms. Hartley have any responsibility to intervene immediately once Ramon shared that he was using marijuana? Why or why not? (**D10**)
8. What legal issues are involved in this case? The student received special education services for an "other health impairment." According to IDEIA Part B (e.g., 34 CFR §300.530), what procedures should be put in place if a long-term suspension or expulsion is being considered for a student with a disability? (**D10**)
9. How did the principal's perception of Ramon as a threat affect this case? Similarly, how did the school's zero tolerance policy affect this case? (**D5, D6, D10**)
10. In this case, there was no mention of parent communication or involvement. How might Ms. Hartley have engaged the family more? (**D7**)

Advanced Applications

1. Use an ethical decision-making model (i.e., Liang et al., 2017) to think about a better course of action that Ms. Hartley should have followed. (**D10**)
2. Research the evidence-based for or against zero tolerance policies and alternatives to suspension and expulsion. What would you recommend based on this research? (**D5, D6**)
3. Role-play a conversation with the principal where you express your concerns and explore alternatives to suspension or expulsion. (**D2**)
4. Review best practices for making manifestation determinations (e.g., Kubick Jr. & Lavik, 2014). Provide recommendations for the school given best practices. (**D10**)
5. Review best practices for threat assessment (e.g., Cornell, 2014). Provide recommendations for the school psychologist to aid the school in determining if Ramon possesses a legitimate threat to the school that would warrant removal. (**D1**)

Case Three: Unacclaimed and Underrepresented

Dr. Esposito recently attended an equity training where she was introduced to data about gifted referral patterns within her district. As the school psychologist, she was alarmed to see that only 2 percent of gifted students at her Title 1 elementary school were Black or Hispanic, despite the school's high percentage of Black and Hispanic students overall (60 percent). This number did not represent the overall demographics of the school population. Additionally, she learned that the gifted rate at this school is 5 percent of the total population compared to another more affluent and predominantly white schools in the district, which was nearly 10 percent. Dr. Esposito noticed the stark disparity both within her school and across the district. She brought this problem back to her school equity team for discussion and review. The team recognized that one issue might be their referral process. A parent or teacher referral in first and second grade was the only point of entry into gifted. They felt this subjective process could be biased and contributing to the disparity. Dr. Esposito reviewed the literature on this issue and pulled ideas from a similar situation presented by Card and Giuliano (2016) and details of how they introduced a universal screening to the process. From her review of the literature, she was amazed at the drastic increase of representation of students of color, specifically Black and Hispanic students, in gifted education after the initiation of a universal screening process.

Like the Card and Giuliano (2016) study, Dr. Esposito was able to institute a new universal screening process at her school. The new procedure included the screening of all second graders using the Naglieri Non-Verbal Ability Test (NNAT), a nonverbal test intended to assess cognitive ability with reduced language demands and culturally bound items. (Naglieri & Ford, 2003). The NNAT was administered by teachers in the second-grade classrooms in under an hour at the end of the first quarter. Dr. Esposito recommended that the school use the same cut-off scores as Card and Giuliano (2016). Students who received a standard score of 130 or higher on the test, and English learner (EL) and Free and Reduced Meals (FARMS) students receiving a standard score of at least 115 on the test, were automatically referred to her school's multidisciplinary team for consideration for a full gifted evaluation and cognitive assessment. The school continued to allow parent and teacher referrals for gifted evaluations.

The aim of the new screening plan was to supplement the pre-existing referral system and boost referral rates for underrepresented groups at her school. Dr. Esposito was pleased to see that the screening program led to similar results as Card and Giuliano (2016). She saw a large increase in the

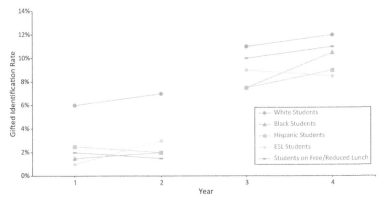

Figure 8.1 Screening Program for Gifted Identification

number of students classified as gifted. The increases specifically included Black, and Hispanic, EL students, as well as students on Free and Reduced Meals. In her inspection of the data, the cognitive assessment scores of the newly identified students were like those identified under the old system. Most of the students of color identified with the new system scored above 130 and did not even require the lower 115 cut-off score. She was able to share this data with her staff. They were surprised and upset to see how many students they had been overlooking with the previous system, but now recognized the importance of committing time and resources to this new system.

Discussion Questions

1. What are the policies and procedures for gifted education referrals in your state or school district? (**D10**)
2. What implications might this have on the representation of diverse groups in the gifted category? (**D8**)
3. How was data-based decision-making critical to equity for diverse populations in this example? (**D1**)
4. In what ways were consultation and collaboration important in this case? What else might have Dr. Esposito had to do from a consultation/collaboration perspective to bring about and maintain this change? (**D2**)
5. How did Dr. Esposito use research to approach this problem? What implications did that have for the outcomes? (**D9**)

Advanced Applications

1. Research evidence-based practices for gifted education. Now that Ms. Esposito has more equitable representation in gifted, what does research say is the best way to provide academic services for this group? (**D3**)
2. Review the Card and Giuliano (2016) article. What organizational principles ended up affecting equitable services? How could the school psychologist serve as an organizational consultant to advocate for a return to the equitable practices? (**D2, O3**)
3. Reflect on the use of cognitive assessments in gifted identification processes. What are the potential issues with the use of cognitive assessments? If they are not utilized, how should gifted students be identified in equitable ways? (**D1, D9**)

Case Four: Transition

Corey, a transgender teen transitioning from female to male, was making the transition to a new neighborhood and a new high school. He had just come out to his parents over the summer and was newly embracing his identity as a transmale. Embarking on the new school, he wanted to change his name from Carol to Corey and his pronoun from "she" to "he" in school records. He also wanted to join the football team. His family was nervous. They wanted to support Corey but were unsure about how he would be received at the new school. They were anxious that it might turn into a major story in the media, after recent similar stories had gone viral. They loved Corey and did not want to see him go through that intense scrutiny. While supportive, Corey's parents themselves were a little uncertain about how to navigate all of this. They were having a hard time with the idea of making the pronoun change. It was a big shift for them.

Given their uncertainty and ambiguity, they asked to meet with someone at the school who could help provide support. The principal put the parents in touch with the school psychologist, Dr. Linnez. Dr. Linnez met with the family the week before school started and she immediately put them at ease. Dr. Linnez informed the family that this school has previous experience supporting transgender teens, given that they have had at least six other transgender students at the school. Upon gaining parent permission and Corey's assent, she shared the name change and preferred pronoun with the staff and front office to change the roster via email.

When school started, Corey's parents attended Back-to-School Night and signed in on the teacher's roster. They were concerned to see that Corey's name was still listed as Carol on the sign-in sheet and that the teacher was not aware of the name change. Later that night, Corey's parents met with the football coach to talk about Corey's interest in joining the junior varsity football team. The coach was open to it but said Corey would have to tell the rest of the team, so they could all be honest as a team about the locker room issue. The parents know that Corey does not feel comfortable with this type of self-disclosure in a public forum and does not want to be "outted" with the team. However, they know that Corey still wants to be on the team. The parents are unsure how to handle this.

Discussion Questions

1. What is the school psychologist's role in helping Corey and his family? Has the school psychologist provided enough support to Corey and his family? Why or why not? (**D10**)
2. Legally, what are the student's rights in this situation? (**D10**)
3. What ethical issues are involved in this case? (**D10**)
4. What consultation and collaboration are needed for the teacher and coaches? (**D2, O5**)
5. What other supports might this student need from the high school? (**D5**)
6. With at least 6 students identifying as transgender, what other supports, services, or professional development might be needed school-wide? (**D7, O5, O6**)
7. What supports might the parents need? What types of resources could the school provide to the parents to navigate their own concerns and needs as they attempt to support Corey? (**D7**)

Advanced Applications

1. Role play the intake conversation with the parents. Have someone take the role of Dr. Linnez, the parents, and Corey. (**D2**)
2. Role play the conversation between the school psychologist and school personnel. Have someone take the role of Dr. Linnez and the coach, the classroom teacher who has the name wrong on the roster. (**D2**)
3. Research community resources in your area for LGBTQ+ students and parents. Create a handout that could be presented to Corey's parents. (**D7**)
4. Dr. Linnez mentioned that the school had practice with transgender teens. What if they did not? What school-wide interventions might be needed to develop a safe climate for LGBTQ+ youth? (**D6**)

5. Dr. Linnez mentioned that there were six transgender teens in the school. What might mental health services look like for those teens as individuals or a group? Research evidence-based approaches for supporting LGBTQ+ teens. (**D4**)
6. The football coach feels that the other players have a right to know that Corey is transgender due to the issue with the shared use of the locker room. Is this accurate? Why or why not? (**D10**)

References

American Psychological Association. (2017a). *Multicultural guidelines: An ecological approach to context, identity, and intersectionality.* www.apa.org/about/policy/multicultural-guidelines

American Psychological Association. (2017b). *Ethical principles of psychologists and code of conduct* (2002, amended effective June 1, 2010, and January 1, 2017). www.apa.org/ethics/code/

Card, D., & Giuliano, L. (2016). Universal screening increases the representation of low-income and minority students in gifted education. *Proceedings of the National Academy of Sciences, 113*(48), 13678–13683. https://doi.org/10.1073/pnas.1605043113

Cornell, D. (2014). Best practices in threat assessment in schools. In P. L. Harrison & A. Thomas (Eds.), *Best practices in school psychology: Systems-level services* (pp. 259–272). National Association of School Psychologists.

Grapin, S. L., & Kranzler, J. H. (2018). *School psychology professional issues and practices.* Springer Publishing Company Individuals with Disabilities Education Improvement Act Part B, 34 CFR §300.530 (2004). https://sites.ed.gov/idea/regs/b/e/300.530

Kubick Jr., R. J., & Lavik, K. B. (2014). Best practices in making manifestation determinations. In P. L. Harrison & A. Thomas (Eds.), *Best practices in school psychology: Student-level services* (pp. 399–414). National Association of School Psychologists.

Liang, B., Chung, A., Diamonti, A. J., Douyon, C. M., Gordon, J. R., Joyner, E. D., Meerkins, T. M., Rene, K. M., Sienkiewicz, S-A., Weber, A., White, A. F., & Wilson, E. S. (2017). Ethical social justice: Do the ends justify the means? *Journal of Community and Applied School Psychology, 27*(4), 298–311. https://doi.org/10.1002/casp.23233

Naglieri, J. A., & Ford, D. Y. (2003). Assessing underrepresentation of gifted minority children using the Naglieri Nonverbal Ability Test (NNAT). *Gifted Child Quarterly, 47*(2), 155–160.

National Association of School Psychologists. (2017). *Strategic plan: 2017–2022.* www.nasponline.org/utility/about-nasp/vision-core-purpose-core-values-and-strategic-goals

National Association of School Psychology. (2020). *The professional standards of the national association of school psychologists.* National Association of School Psychologists.

Understanding Research and Evidence-Based Practice 9

Domain 9: Research and Evidence-Based Practice

"School psychologists have knowledge of research design, statistics, measurement, and varied data collection and analysis techniques sufficient for understanding research, interpreting data, and evaluating programs in applied settings. As scientist practitioners, school psychologists evaluate and apply research as a foundation for service delivery and, in collaboration with others, use various techniques and technology resources for data collection, measurement, and analysis to support effective practices at the individual, group, and/or systems levels." (NASP, 2020, p. 9)

According to the NASP *Principles of Professional Ethics* (NASP, 2020), school psychologists are committed to both "responsible assessment and intervention practices" guided by research and evidence-based practice (NASP, 2020, p. 46) and "contributing to the school psychology knowledge base" (NASP, 2020, p. 55). The four cases presented within this chapter highlight some of the ways that school psychologists utilize research and evidence-based practice to provide school psychological services.

First, as practicing school psychologists, it is important for school psychologists to be ethical consumers of research (Keith, 2008). By upholding our professional standard of "continuing professional development" (NASP, 2020, p. 45) and staying engaged with the latest research through memberships in professional organizations and consistent reading of the latest research in the field, school psychologists can ensure that they are applying the most up-to-date research in their practices within schools. Case one, "The Case for Effective Instruction," allows for discussion of the research to practice gap in education and how to uphold our ethical standard to seek "interventions described in peer-reviewed professional research literature and found to be efficacious," (NASP, 2020, p. 47) in order to become a better advocate for the science of reading practices within schools. Practicing school psychologists must be effective consumers of instruction and intervention research and this case allows for discussion of how to ensure that this is a reality in practice.

School psychologists can distribute their knowledge about research and evidence-based practice to advocate for best practices (Keith, 2008). There is an ongoing need in schools to advocate for effective practices in curriculum, instruction, social-emotional and behavioral supports, family-school relationships and more to assure the best outcomes possible for individual students. School psychologists can apply their knowledge of evidence-based practice at the district, school-wide, and class-wide level.

At the individual student level, school psychologists ensure that interventions selected to assist a child are evidence-based, are implemented with integrity, and are evaluated to determine their effectiveness. School psychologists can assist with the ongoing progress monitoring of interventions as well as the evaluations of interventions to determine their effectiveness or the need for adjustments to ensure better outcomes. The school psychologist should work with fellow team members to ensure that decision-making occurs from a data-based approach. Case two "Evaluating Intervention Integrity," focuses on how data must be analyzed to determine the potential reasons for inadequate progress of interventions. In this case, there is opportunity for discussion about how to ensure intervention integrity and what types of data should be collected and analyzed to ensure that decision-making processes are utilized based on interventions that have been implemented as intended.

At the class-wide and school-wide level, school psychologists apply similar strategies to evaluate needs, select evidence-based interventions, and monitor the progress of interventions to assist with class-wide and/or school-based functioning. School psychologists are also able to create and disseminate needs assessments to better understand the needs of the staff, students, families or other stakeholders within the community or school district. The third case, "The Time Crunch," provides opportunities for discussion about how the best intentions might cause ethical and professional issues when assessments are selected without proper due diligence to ensure that they are appropriate for use with a specific population. School psychologists have an ethical obligation to ensure assessment techniques adhere to "responsible, research-based practice" (NASP, 2020, p. 46).

School psychologists can be conductors of research or program evaluation to assist in educational decision-making (Keith, 2008) and should contribute to the school psychology knowledge base by conducting research (NASP, 2020). School psychologists have the knowledge to be key members of school and district-wide teams that seek to utilize data to make programmatic improvements. The fourth case, "Evaluating School-Wide Programs," tackles this issue and demonstrates how school psychologists can assist schools in creating and managing the program evaluation of school-wide programs.

Case One: The Case for Effective Instruction

The school psychologist at Jefferson Elementary School, Ms. Johnson, is noticing a pattern in her school's special education referrals. For the third year in a row, she has conducted at least sixty evaluations based on referrals for concerns about specific learning disability (SLD) in reading. Many parents come in with concerns that their child might be dyslexic. There is a strong parent advocacy group in the region that has been informing parents about dyslexia, so parents are alarmed that their child is missing an important diagnosis along with the services that the school should be provided for children with disabilities. Most of the students in third through fifth grade that Ms. Johnson evaluates for a specific learning disability in reading do end up qualifying in the area of reading, with significant discrepancies in word-level reading, pseudoword (nonsense word) reading, and basic reading. She wonders why there is seemingly such a large percentage of children with reading difficulties in her district and decides to investigate further to look for trends in the data. Specifically, she looks more closely at her primary-grade curriculum-based measurement benchmark screening data and notices that the students are mostly on grade-level and around the 50th percentile upon entry to kindergarten, 80 percent are progressing appropriately according to the classification system in her benchmarking data (see Figure 9.1), but by the end of first grade, only 60 percent of students are on-level, while 30 percent of student are below level in the targeted level, and 10 percent are in the intensive needs coding level (see Figure 9.2).

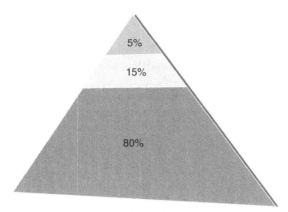

Figure 9.1 Kindergarten Benchmark Reading Screening Data

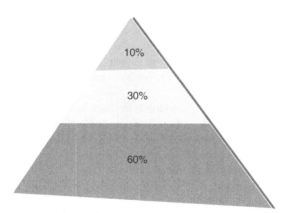

Figure 9.2 First-Grade Benchmark Reading Screening Data

Ms. Johnson recently attended a webinar about the science of reading. In this webinar, the presenter talked about dyslexia as a potential curriculum and instruction problem. The presenter used the term *dystaughtia* to make that point clear. In the training, Ms. Johnson learned the difference between balanced literacy and structured literacy as well as the potential problems with whole-language instruction, or guided reading approaches especially for students who benefit from more explicit phonics instruction. When Ms. Johnson returned to her school, she started inquiring more about the primary reading curriculum and intervention programs.

She spent time observing reading instruction in classrooms. She observed teachers prompting students to "look at the picture" to decode unknown words as opposed to teaching specific word analysis patterns. Upon further research, Ms. Johnson discovered that the school was not using scientifically based reading curriculum or intervention programs in the primary grades. In fact, the curriculum and intervention programs they were using were being explicitly criticized in the scientific reading literature. She started to gather information on explicit phonics-based curriculum and interventions that have a solid evidence base.

Discussion Questions

1. How did Ms. Johnson become an avid consumer of research and how did this help inform her practices at the school? **(D9)**
2. Why is it important for a school psychologist to continue attending trainings and professional development sessions, reviewing scholarly research, and utilizing evidence-based intervention clearinghouses? **(D9, O6)**
3. What data did Ms. Johnson use to help analyze this problem? What other data might be helpful to analyze this problem further and plan solutions? **(D1)**
4. Ms. Johnson is primarily working in isolation as she comes to these realizations, other than her observations and interviews. How might this be problematic? What should she do to involve and empower others in her problem-identification, analysis, and search for solutions? Which key stakeholders should be involved? **(D2, O4, O5)**
5. What implications could her research have for academic services and outcomes at the school? **(D3)**
6. How will her shift from evaluating individual students to looking at this problem with a systems-level school-wide lens affect student and staff outcomes? Her time/role in the school? **(D5)**
7. What other data might she need to explore potential equity issues that might also be present in her referral patterns? **(D1, D8)**
8. What is the school psychologist's role regarding decisions around curriculum and instruction? **(D3, D5)**
9. What are the legal criteria for an SLD reading qualification in your state/district? How can you apply that definition to this case? **(D1, D9)**
10. How is her research an important step in legal and ethical decision-making? (competence, making decisions about ruling out the lack of appropriate instruction) **(D10)**

Advanced Applications

1. Ms. Johnson indicated that she did some research to find out that the school may not be applying best practices in reading instruction and effective Tier III interventions. What are some sources that school psychologists might want to use to conduct such research? Create a chart of options for exploring resources that might be readily available to all practicing school psychologists. (**D3, D9**)

2. Research some of the programs and approaches to reading instruction that are mentioned in the case. What are research findings on some of these approaches (balanced literacy, whole-language instruction, guided reading)? (**D3**)

3. Select an area of reading to research and present your findings to the group. (**D3**)

4. Within the academic and educational community, there have been specific concerns that the science of reading is not effectively or adequately applied within schools. What are some reasons for this "research to practice gap"? What are some strategies that a school can use to ensure the application of the science of reading into their curriculum, instruction, and training practices? (**D3, D5, D9**)

Case Two: Evaluating Intervention Integrity

Sara, the school psychologist at Cedar Grove Elementary School, was very involved with the tiered problem-solving teams at the school. She collected data for all students in K-2 who were receiving Tier III math interventions. At this school, Tier III math interventions consisted of 30 minutes, twice per week, of intensive math instruction on pre-identified areas of need based on ongoing math screening assessments. She set up a plan to monitor student progress for all students at the Tier III level. These data were collected monthly throughout the school year. At the end of three months, Sara was dismayed to find out that there were limited to no positive results in the progress of these students. In fact, only 18–22 percent of these children made adequate progress (see Table 9.1). She presented this data to the team, that the students in general were not making progress, and recommended referrals for special education evaluation for most of the children in Tier III. The team agreed to meet about some of the students, beginning with those who have shown no progress.

Table **9.1** Tier III Intervention Progress Monitoring Data: Percentage of Students Meeting Individual Goals for Math

Month	Kindergarten Students	First-Grade Students	Second-Grade Students
September	16%	18%	17%
October	16%	19%	18%
November	18%	22%	20%

At the first meeting to discuss the data on one of the children, the teacher reported that the student had not made progress in Tier III, but then in passing comments that she did not know how often the Tier III intervention was supposed to take place and that maybe the student should just get more intervention time. This led to a discussion of the Tier III plan and whether this plan was implemented as intended. It was determined that the student had not received the intervention as intended. Specifically, the ongoing math screening assessments were not routinely given to understand areas of need for targeted instruction. In the ensuing discussions, the teachers indicated that they did not feel like they had the time to do what was being asked of them and reported that often the plans were not discussed with then in advance. The teachers reported a great deal of frustration at the lack of communication. Sara left this meeting concerned that teachers were ready to give up on providing math-based interventions for students who needed additional support. She was not sure what should be the next steps in tackling this school-based issue.

Discussion Questions

1. Are the data presented, sufficient for understanding happened with Tier III math instruction at the school? What were the flaws with this evaluation approach? (**D1, D9**)
2. What other data should have been collected and analyzed in conjunction with the student progress monitoring? (**D1, D9**)
3. What should be the next steps for this team? (**D3, D10**)
4. What should the school psychologist do in terms of consultation and collaboration for this case and other similar cases moving forward? (**D2**)

5. What are potential needs related to the professional development of staff within the building? What skills might be needed to better implement planned instruction? (**D5, O6**)
6. The teachers report frustrations about the perceived lack of communication about these intervention plans. What might have gone wrong here and how can this be improved? (**O4**)

Advanced Applications

1. Research an intervention for math that might be used for early numeracy intervention at the Tier III level. Once you have selected the intervention, create an intervention script for a teacher utilizing this intervention. (**D1, D3, D9**)
2. Using the intervention strategy selected for question 1, list some options for how the school psychologist might monitor the implementation of this intervention. (**D1, D2, D3, D9**)
3. Create an implementation fidelity checklist for the teacher (self-evaluation) and for the school psychologist (class observation) to utilize. (**D1, D2, D3, D9**)
4. This case focused on Tier III interventions. However, given the problems noted with effective implementation integrity, what additional suggestions do you have for the team in terms of ensuring appropriate Tier I and Tier II intervention implementation. (**D2, D3**)

Case Three: The Time Crunch

During the professional development sessions for educators two days before the beginning of the school year, the new Director of Student Services at a large school district in New Mexico informed the student support staff that she would like to begin implementing a school-wide depression screening for all students from fourth grade to twelfth grade. In this school, 60 percent of students are English learners. She wanted all students to be screened by the end of the first month of school so the data could be used to provide tiered social-emotional support for students who were experiencing depression or other mental health concerns. She asked the school counseling and school psychology staff to select a depression screener that could be purchased right away so screening could start early in the school year.

The team was overwhelmed with other back-to-school tasks and was not able to meet to discuss the many different possibilities of screeners available until the second week of school. Prior to that meeting, the director reiterated that she wanted the screening process to start immediately, and the team felt the pressure of these time constraints. Even worse, during the meeting to discuss various screeners, multiple members of the team were called out of the meeting room to deal with various issues. By the end of the meeting, the school counselor suggested selecting the one screener that she was aware of because she had recently received marketing material from a publishing company about this new screener. The team agreed that they should order that screener and the large-scale purchase was made. Unfortunately, the team did not spend any time discussing the process that they will use to assist students who are identified with the screener as needing support due to depressive symptoms and/or suicidal ideation. They also did not discuss how, when, or who will intervene based on the results of the screening.

When the screener arrives, the school psychologist took time to read through the entire manual. She was dismayed as she realized several critical problems with the screener that had been purchased. She realized that the screener was designed for middle and high school. Therefore, it cannot be administered to the fourth and fifth grade students as requested by the Director of Student Services. Further, she was concerned that the norm group did not adequately represent students of color, particularly Black students. The norm group also appeared to lack representation from certain areas of the United States. Most children in the norm group lived in the North East area of the United States, not representative of New Mexico. Lastly, she had concerns about the practicality of the test, since there was a larger amount of test items than expected and many of the test items appeared to be written at an advanced reading level. Given that the school population included 40 percent of students served in the EL program, the school psychologist was concerned that they may have difficulty understanding the test questions.

Discussion Questions

1. What are the issues involved with the selection of this depression screener? (**D1, D9, D10**)
2. What are the cornerstones of measurement that should have all been evaluated prior to the selection of the depression screener? (**D9**)

3. What process should the team have engaged in instead of what happened in this case? (**D1, D2**)
4. This case highlights the concept of "if you screen, you must intervene." What is meant by this concept? (**D4**)
5. Given that the team did not have the time to adequately research the selection of the screener, it seems unlikely that they will have the necessary time to devote themselves to intervention. How did the team not adequately plan for the intervention piece of this process? What should have been done differently to ensure a plan for intervention based on screening results? (**D10**)
6. Keith (2008) discusses the issue of access to research as a potential barrier for school psychologists in being effective consumers of research. What are ways to increase access to research as practicing school psychologists? What avenues should be explored to ensure consistent access to up-to-date best practices? (**D9**)
7. What potential concerns related to the use of this screener exist regarding the large percentage of EL students at this school? Has the school done enough to consider their ability to access this screener? What else should be done? (**D8**)

Advanced Applications

1. Review the research on depression screeners. Select a screening tool to suggest to this team given the concerns listed. Critically review the screener that you have selected. What are the advantages and limitations of the screener that you selected? (**D1, D9**)
2. If the school team analyzes the results of the depression screening and finds that many students are expressing that they have feelings of depression and/or may be at risk for suicidal ideation, what should happen next? What should be immediate and long-term next steps for interactions with students who have indicated these concerns? (**D4, D6**)
3. If the results suggest that there are many students who are at risk for depression and/or suicidal ideation, what might this say about the school climate? Are there school-wide programs that should be considered? Research school-wide programming designed for social-emotional learning and present some options for implementation. What are the strengths and limitations of such programs? (**D4, D5, D6**).

Case Four: Evaluating School-Wide Programs

Janice is a new school psychologist who has just started her first job as a school psychologist at a large, suburban middle school serving children in 6–8 grade. The school has approximately 900 students (approximately 300 students per grade). When starting this job, she was thrilled to learn that the school reported that they were using restorative practices (RP) to deal with student misbehaviors and discipline. While it was mentioned in her new employee orientation as well as the first meetings prior to the beginning of school by the school principal, she did not get many details about the practices that were in place in the school. Since she had just completed graduate school, she had a lot of updated information about the potential benefits of utilizing restorative practices as opposed to zero-tolerance policies for handling discipline in schools. When asking some of her co-workers about the restorative practices program, she found that some were very enthusiastic about it and felt strongly that it had "worked" in reducing punitive disciplinary measures in the school and by extension creating a more positive teacher-student relationships since it was implemented two years ago. However, other staff seemed to know little about the program or felt that the program was a way for students to "get away" with misbehaviors. According to Fronius et al. (2019), many schools may be utilizing Restorative Justice principles or "restorative practices" in different ways, with no universal application of restorative practices within schools. Janice felt that this was happening at her new school.

While hesitant to question the procedures in place as a new school psychologist, Janice decided to approach the school principal in mid-October and asked about the specifics about the plan that was in place, what efforts (if any) had been made to document its effectiveness, and whether there was a team/person who was involved in ongoing monitoring and program evaluation of this program to make any necessary improvements. The principal was open to a discussion of these questions and was impressed with Janice's seemingly advanced knowledge about these concepts and school-wide problem-solving. By the end of the meeting, she told Janice that these things were not being done, but she would really like someone to do them. She asked Janice if she would be willing to lead a team that would serve to evaluate the program in place. Janice, a bit taken-aback by this request, nonetheless felt that she had no choice but to agree to take the lead on this. While she was thrilled that so much trust had been granted her as a brand-new school psychologist and was very interested in assisting to ensure the success of this program that she believed could be successful at this school, she was very overwhelmed about what her first steps should be to establish a team and begin an evaluation of this program at a school-wide level.

According to Fronius et al. (2019), future research is needed regarding the necessary factors related to a school's readiness to implement RP as well as how to establish a clear and largely acceptable definition of RP. Further, additional outcome data are necessary in schools that are implementing RP successfully so that replication is possible. Janice created and distributed a survey to staff regarding their knowledge and need for training in the policies/procedures and philosophies related to restorative practices. Results of the survey, which used a Likert scale (1=Agree; 2=Neither Agree/Disagree (Neutral); 3=Disagree), are reported in Table 9.2. Janice also researched and compiled data on both in-school and out-of-school suspensions for the past three years (Year 1=prior to implementation; Year 2=initial year of implementation; Year 3=second year of implementation). The results are presented in Table 9.3 and Figure 9.3 and suggested to Janice that the first year of implementation of the program may have been more successful than the second year, which was the year before she started at the school. Beyond these two pieces of information, Janice realized that she needed more support in creating a comprehensive program evaluation plan. She emailed staff to find volunteers to create a committee and received responses from four teacher volunteers. She set a meeting up for the following week.

Table 9.2 Faculty Survey About Restorative Practices Implementation

Survey Question	Percent Agree	Percent Neutral	Percent Disagree
I have sufficient knowledge about the philosophy behind Restorative Practices.	40%	15%	45%
I have received sufficient training about how our school employs Restorative Practices.	40%	10%	50%
Our school has ongoing support/training to implement restorative practices in our school.	10%	15%	75%
I believe that there has been a noticeable change in our school climate since implementing Restorative Practices.	35%	40%	25%

Table 9.3 Impact of Restorative Practices: Number of Suspensions

	Number of Out-of-School Suspensions by Grade	Number of In-School Suspensions by Grade
Year 1 (baseline)	6th Grade: 18	6th Grade: 45
	7th Grade: 24	7th Grade: 40
	8th Grade: 41	8th Grade: 60
Year 2 (1st Year of Implementation)	6th Grade: 5	6th Grade: 22
	7th Grade: 12	7th Grade: 30
	8th Grade: 17	8th Grade: 36
Year 3 (2nd Year of Implementation	6th Grade: 12	6th Grade: 38
	7th Grade: 20	7th Grade: 40
	8th Grade: 28	8th Grade: 49

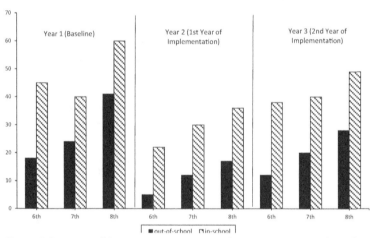

Figure 9.3 Impact of Restorative Practices Implementation on Number of Suspensions

Discussion Questions

1. What is the rationale behind implementing restorative practices? (**D5, D6**)
2. The case mentions zero tolerance policies. What is meant by zero tolerance policies? Why is the use of zero tolerance policies in schools an area of concern? (**D5**)

3. What are some initial concerns regarding the implementation of this program at the middle school? (**D5**)
4. Janice agrees to lead the program evaluation of this program. What would you suggest that she do first in terms of engaging stakeholders to create a team to work with her? How can she ensure that she has a collaborative team to work with on the evaluation? (**D2**)
5. Janice has some initial data regarding the program that she presented. Discuss what this data demonstrates. What do we know so far based on this data? (**D9**)
6. The principal of this school was very receptive for additional assistance in the implementation and evaluation of this program. However, she may not have adequately estimated the amount of time or resources for Janice to work on a major project like this with her daily responsibilities. How can school psychologists advocate for adequate time to engage in school-wide projects, such as this program evaluation? (**O3**)

Advanced Applications

1. Based on your understanding of implementation science, what types of ongoing evaluations should be put into place to begin to evaluate this school-wide program? (**D9**)
2. Create a plan for the program evaluation that this committee could implement to evaluate the effectiveness of RJ at this school. (**D9**)
3. Create a training and ongoing coaching plan for the sustainable implementation of this program for future years. (**D2, D5, D9, D10**)
4. As indicated in this case, there are many variations of models related to restorative practices. Research the various models and their evidence base. (**D9**)

References

Fronius, T., Darling-Hammond, S., Persson, H., Guckenburg, S., Hurley, N., & Petrosino, A. (2019). *Restorative justice in U.S. schools: An updated research review*. WestEd Justice & Prevention Research Center.

Keith, T. Z. (2008). Best practices in using and conducting research in applied settings. In A. Thomas & J. Grimes (Eds.), *Best practices in school psychology V* (5th ed., pp. 2165–2175). National Association of School Psychologists.

National Association of School Psychology. (2020). *The professional standards of the national association of school psychologists*. National Association of School Psychologists.

Understanding Legal, Ethical, and Professional Practice

10

Domain 10: Legal, Ethical, and Professional Practice

"School psychologists have knowledge of the history and foundations of school psychology; multiple service models and methods; ethical, legal, and professional standards; and other factors related to professional identity and effective practice as school psychologists. School psychologists provide services consistent with ethical, legal, and professional standards; engage in responsive ethical and professional decision-making; collaborate with other professionals; and apply professional work characteristics needed for effective practice as school psychologists, including effective interpersonal skills, responsibility, adaptability, initiative, dependability, technological competence, advocacy skills, respect for human diversity, and a commitment to social justice and equity." (NASP, 2020, p. 10)

The practice of school psychology is driven by federal, state, and local laws and regulations (e.g., IDEIA, 2004; FERPA, 1974; Section 504 of the Rehabilitation Act, 1973), ethical guidelines (NASP-PPE, 2020), multicultural guidelines (APA, 2017a), and professional standards (e.g., NASP, 2020; APA, 2017b).

Domain 10 highlights the fact that school psychologists must always practice in ways that are consistent with ethical, professional, and legal standards. This domain also focuses on the necessity for school psychologists to actively engage with professional resources, collaborate with other professionals, and seek out professional development opportunities to stay abreast in the latest standards for best practice within the field. School psychologists also should, whenever possible, support the next generation of practitioners by providing mentorship and supervision of graduate students in school psychology and engage with the profession of school psychology.

It is an ethical responsibility for school psychologists to ensure that evidence-based practices, which are in line with federal and state laws, are implemented in schools to best support the children in need of intervention, accommodations, and other types of support to be successful in their academic, social, emotional, and behavioral development. The first case emphasizes the importance of ethical decision-making when a school psychologist is confronted with a colleague who may be making decisions and operating in a manner that could be harmful to children. Case three also highlights a common dilemma that school psychologists might confront when they are asked to practice outside of their knowledge base or expertise, albeit in the name of helping children. These cases will illustrate ethical guidelines of competence (NASP-PPE, II.1), non-maleficence (American Psychological Association, 2017b), and priority of child welfare (NASP, 2020).

School psychologists must be knowledgeable in all relevant educational and psychological standards of ethical behavior, as well as the legal standards and guidelines governing educational and school psychological practice at the federal, state, and local jurisdictions in which they work. Case Two raises issues surrounding the type of information that is shared about children and their families in schools and how to make determinations about the necessity of sharing specific types of information. This case discussion will allow for reflection upon FERPA (1974) and NASP-PPE guiding principles of privacy and confidentiality (NASP, 2020). The fourth case, "Applying Law to Practice," presents a specific situation in which a school team must decide how to apply applicable laws, including the application of guidelines for 504 eligibility, to best serve the needs of a student with a chronic health concern. School psychologists have an ethical obligation to "respect laws pertinent to the practice of school psychology" to choose the correct course of action (NASP, 2020, p. 54). This case will allow for practice of that principle.

The cases in this chapter highlight just a few of the various types of situations that school psychologists might be called on to navigate to ensure appropriate ethical, legal, and professional practice within the profession of school psychology. While it is not possible to include the full range of the types of legal and ethical issues that school psychologists must understand with just four case presentations, the cases represent a sampling of common issues that school psychologists might confront while working in schools.

Case One: Colleague Indiscretions

Laurie, a first-year school psychologist who identifies as White, worked in a large, urban school district in a major United States city. She was assigned to four different school buildings in the district, so she only spent approximately one day per week in each school. Most of the students and staff at all her schools identified as Black. Because she was assigned to four schools, Laurie had not been able to develop many relationships with staff or students in any of her buildings thus far.

One day in October while Laurie was in her office completing paperwork, a middle school student left his classroom and came to Laurie's office crying. He said that his teacher had pushed him. Apparently, the teacher was charging his phone and the student tripped over the cord, which pulled the phone to the ground and broke the screen. The student indicated that he had tripped over the charger accidentally, although he admitted that he had been out of his seat at the time when he was supposed to be at his desk completing an assignment. The teacher's reaction to seeing his phone break was to push the student away from the phone. The student indicated that the push was hard enough to make him stumble backwards onto the floor. Laurie spent time assisting the student to calm down and the student stayed in her office until the bell rang for the next class. He then left for his next period class. Laurie sat in her office wondering what she should do next. She thought that she should report this incident to the school administration, but she was new to working at this school building. She did not have a good understanding of the context of the classroom or the incident. She also did not know the teacher or this student well, so she had no background information about whether this report from the student was credible.

Upon further reflection, Laurie decided to report the incident for investigation and left her office to attempt to find the building principal. Unfortunately, the principal was out of the building at a meeting for the day. Therefore, Laurie found one of the assistant principals (APs) and discussed the situation with that administrator. Laurie suggested to the AP that perhaps she should pull a few students from the class to document what they might have seen regarding this incident. The AP told Laurie that she "will handle it from here" so Laurie went back to her office to complete her day of work with other tasks. The following day, Laurie was called into the principal's office and reprimanded for suggesting to her AP the previous day that there should be a report on this incident. The principal says, "If we reported every instance like this, we wouldn't have any teachers left."

Laurie left the principal's office confused and disheartened. She considered filing a report up the chain of command about the administrative team's lack of response. However, she decided that it was best to try to create relationships with these new colleagues, so she decided not to do anything. Laurie also knew that each principal was involved in her annual evaluation and therefore did not want to risk having a poor evaluation from this principal by escalating the situation further. The school psychologists in this district were evaluated using the same evaluation tools that were used to evaluate teachers and the principal of each building had significant input into the evaluation. As an untenured school psychologist, she feared that she risked a negative evaluation if she pursued this situation further. She never heard that this situation was ever investigated. The student who reported the incident to Laurie never sought her out for assistance for the remainder of the school year.

Discussion Questions

1. What are the ethical issues associated with this situation? Use the APA Code of Ethics (American Psychological Association, 2017b) and the NASP Principles for Professional Ethics (2020) to guide your discussion. (**D10**)
2. What are the potential legal issues associated with this case? Research the mandatory reporting laws in your state and policies in your school district(s) to assist in answering this question. (**D10**)
3. What are some different choices that Laurie should have considered in this situation? Apply an ethical decision-making model (e.g., Liang et al., 2017) to this dilemma. (**D10**)
4. Discuss the difficulties involved with establishing professional relationships as a school psychologist when assigned to multiple buildings. How might this lack of relationships have influenced what occurred in this situation? (**D2, O4**)
5. When the principal indicates that "if we reported every instance like this, we wouldn't have any teachers left," what potential system-wide issues does this signal for the school as a whole? What might the school psychologist need to do to follow up on this potential school-wide issue? (**D4, D5, D6, O2, O4**)

6. What are the social justice and equity issues that might be occurring in this case? What are the potential social power differences at play regarding race and gender and how might these factors influence how each participant reacted? (**D8**)

7. Laurie was concerned because the principal is involved in her annual evaluation. Skalski and Myers (2014) advocate for using the NASP Practice Model as a basis for the evaluation of school psychologists. How might using the teacher evaluation tool potentially negatively impact school psychologists in general (and Laurie in this specific case)? (**D10, O1**)

8. Why might the student not have returned to Laurie for further assistance? (**D4**)

Advanced Applications

1. It seems clear that there are potential issues with the school climate in this school. Research best practices on how school climate can be evaluated. (**O2, D1, D6, D9**)

2. In this case, the principal alludes to the idea that teachers utilize punitive measures as a disciplinary tactic. Assuming a thorough needs assessment revealed that positive classroom management is a need within this school, what evidenced-based interventions could be considered to develop positive classrooms? (**D5, D6, D9**)

3. Role play a conversation between the principal and Laurie. (**D2**)

4. Research models of evaluation for school psychologists. What should be incorporated into these evaluations? Who should ideally evaluate school psychologists within school systems? (**O1, D10**)

Case Two: Idle Gossip vs. Professional Information: Can You Tell the Difference?

Jackie, a school psychologist, was recently transferred within her district from the high school level to one of the district's middle schools in the spring of the school year. Within her first few weeks working at her new placement, she received a new case with an incoming middle school student with counseling services written in her IEP. The school psychologist participated in the transition meeting with the team from the elementary school in May and the counseling goal was put in place to continue in middle school. Jackie was designated as the person to provide counseling for this student.

Over the summer, Jackie ran into the elementary-level school psychologist, Kathy, at a local conference. Over lunch with several other professionals who were attending the conference from various school districts, the elementary-level school psychologist, Kathy, told Jackie about some of the children transitioning to her middle school in the Fall. She told stories about the various families, gave a great deal of information about this child on Jackie's counseling caseload. She jokingly said, "that family is a nightmare." Jackie was intrigued and asked Kathy for more details, Kathy said, "just look them up online! You'll see!" The other educators at the table laughed at this comment and began telling stories about some of the children and families from their own schools. That evening, Jackie searched Google with the family's last name. She found information about the arrest of the adult-aged older brother for selling drugs. She also found arrest records for the father's past drug use and for car thefts. Finally, she found multiple posts on the mother's Facebook page about these "unfair" arrests and how her family was being targeted by the police.

When school started in the fall, Jackie shared the information that she found online with the student's seven teachers, so they understood the family life of their incoming student. Maria, the school counselor, expresses alarm that the teachers were all provided with this information. Jackie argued to Maria that she had shared this information with all the teachers to increase their empathy and compassion for the child when working with him. She also felt that since the information was readily available online, she had not violated any confidentiality of the student or the family.

Discussion Questions

1. What are the ethical issues involved in this situation? What are the potential legal issues? (**D10**)
2. Should a school psychologist search for information online about a family/child for the stated goal of being better able to serve that child and his/her specific needs? Why or why not? What are the benefits and consequences? What are the potential ethical issues associated with this? (**D10**)
3. In Harris and Robinson Kurpius's (2014) study, they report that one-third of 315 counseling and psychology graduate students surveyed the internet to find information about a client. They recommend graduate students need to examine the purpose that an online disclosure is serving and whether there is a potential to cause harm to the client. What would

be the potential need for disclosure in this situation (if any)? What is the potential harm? (**D10**)

4. What does the NASP (2020) Principles of Professional Ethics say in terms of seeking information on a client that is not disclosed in sessions? Do clients have the right to control what information is disclosed to a psychologist? (**D10**)

5. How can a school psychologist differentiate between necessary information to assist a child and gossip about a family/child? In the case, what types of information would you consider "gossip"? Which information is important for the psychologist to know? The teachers? (**D10**)

6. What does the NASP (2020) Principles of Professional Ethics advise in terms of what to do if you suspect another school psychologist colleague has crossed ethical boundaries? (**D10**)

7. Ethical issues aside, how do the lunch table conversations reflect assumptions and beliefs about the family or other similar families? What issues does this raise in terms of school staff relationships with families? (**D7, O2**)

Advanced Applications

1. How would you respond, in this scenario, if you were the school counselor, Maria, who worked with Jackie? Apply an ethical decision-making model (e.g., Williams et al., 2008) to this situation. (**D10**)

2. Role play a conversation between two mental health professionals in this scenario (e.g., Kathy and Jackie, or Jackie and Maria). Practice how you might respond if someone shares gossip with you or private information that they have looked up online. (**D2, D10, O4**)

3. It sounds as if the family could use some support, what might be your next steps if you were Jackie and were truly concerned about the family? Role play a parent phone call and initial interview. (**D7**)

Case Three: Jack of All Trades?

Christina is a 16-year-old White junior. She attends a regional high school located in a rural area. Students attend this high school from a large radius, approximately 30 miles, given the rural nature of the area. Over the past several months, Christina's teachers and the school nurse have expressed concern that Christina has lost a great deal of weight. The school nurse called home to the parents after the yearly nurse screening to report that she had lost 27 pounds since the previous year's screening in which she was of average weight. The nurse further indicated concern that she appeared significantly underweight. At the time of that phone call, the parents also indicated concern about Christina losing weight rapidly to the nurse. They indicated that she had begun a diet several months before to lose 10 pounds and that she has since become "obsessed" with tracking calories and exercising. The parents reported significant family conflicts, particularly during family mealtimes, because Christina will often refuse to eat. Christina's mother indicated that this was causing a great deal of stress in the family and indicated that she would be seeking out professional help for her daughter.

Three weeks later, the mother called the school psychologist, Denise, and indicated that she had not found any local counseling resources that specialized in eating disorders. She said the closest counselor was 110 miles away from their house. Christina's mother was greatly distressed that she could not find support in the community for Christina and said it was just not feasible for the family to take her to a counselor 110 miles away. The mother asked Denise if she would begin counseling with Christina during school hours with the goal of helping to resolve some of her issues surrounding her weight and eating. Denise was reluctant to agree to do this. During her training program, she did not receive any specific training on working with adolescents with eating disorders. However, since it was clear that there were limited options in the area and that Christina would not get help in this area without school-based support, Denise agreed to begin counseling immediately. That evening Denise searched treatment approaches for use with adolescents with eating disorders and started counseling Christina the next day.

Discussion Questions

1. What are the potential ethical issues involved in this situation? (**D10**)
2. How can the NASP Principles for Professional Ethics (2020) help guide decision-making in this situation? (**D10**)
3. What are potential avenues that the school psychologist might need to explore to aid Christina? (**D4, D7**)
4. What family and community-based resources could be explored to assist in a situation like this? (**D7**)
5. Should the school psychologist engage in school-based counseling with Christina? Why or why not? (**D7**)

6. In what ways, could Christina and the school nurse collaborate to offer support for Christina in school while not offering actual treatment for a potential eating disorder? (**D2**)

7. How can school psychologists continually engage in professional development as practicing professionals to ensure that they continue to develop skills? Where should they seek out training opportunities, particularly if they do not live in an area with many trainings available? (**O6**)

Advanced Applications

1. Research evidence-based interventions or approaches to working with teens with eating disorders. What training is required to develop competency in those approaches? (**D4, D10**)

2. Gather resources in your own area for eating disorder support (e.g., counselors with specialty, clinics, support groups). Create a handout for parents and/or teens. (**D4, D7**)

3. Beebe-Frankenberger and Goforth (2014) discuss this issue of lack of access to external resources with specific types of expertise. They also discuss how lack of public transportation can limit families' ability to access these limited outside resources. They suggest telehealth as a potential solution to the challenges of access to services and specialized expertise. Research the emerging use of telehealth resources and discuss how it can be applied in rural settings. (**D2, D4, D10**)

Case Four: Applying Law to Practice

Jessica, a Black fifth-grade student at Jackson Elementary School has always been a high honor roll student in the school; in fact, she earned all As in all classes since enrolling in school as a Kindergarten student. Her teachers' report card comments throughout the years included high praise for her advanced academic performance, her leadership skills, and positive prosocial skills. Her state-generated standardized test scores have consistently been in the top five to 10 percent of all performers in the state in both language arts and math. All teachers throughout her school years indicated that she performed well above her grade level in all academic areas.

In the beginning of fourth grade, the school community was dismayed to learn that Jessica had been diagnosed with leukemia over the summer. Her parents called the school to inform them that she would not be starting the year in school and requested a home instruction arrangement. The school arranged home schooling, which allowed Jessica to continue with her academic progress while undergoing intensive treatment for leukemia. Throughout fourth grade, Jessica had cycles of chemotherapy that required her to stay in the hospital. However, in between cycles, she engaged in home instruction and the teacher indicated at the end of the year that she had done quite well with fourth grade academic material.

In fifth grade, Jessica was officially in remission and returned to school full-time. While she still missed some days of school for check-ups with various doctors, she was mostly able to attend school. After the first quarter, Jessica's mother called the school to ask about the possibility of a 504 Plan for Jessica. Her first quarter grades were mostly Bs and Jessica's mother was very concerned that this represented a change in her performance from her performance prior to her diagnosis and year-long chemotherapy treatments. At a meeting to discuss this issue, her mother provided documents from Jessica's oncologist that discussed the potential long-term impact on functioning for children throughout and after the treatment process. However, the 504 Team, including Jessica's current fifth grade teacher, all indicated that they felt that Jessica was doing fine academically and did not need further accommodations. The fifth-grade teacher reported that Jessica was functioning on grade level in all subject areas and indicated to Jessica's mother that she should be pleased that her daughter is earning Bs in all classes, since other children in her class have done much worse in the first quarter of fifth grade. In short, the school team did not believe that there was an academic impact. The meeting was tension-filled. Jessica's mother cried at one point and said she did not feel the team was listening to her concerns. The meeting ended without a decision about whether Jessica qualified for a 504 Plan; although the team indicated that they would conduct some research into the matter and contact the mother in approximately one week. The school psychologist was interested in the information that the mother provided from the oncologist regarding the potential of long-term academic impacts in functioning for children after treatment for cancer and was interested in learning more from the oncologist. However, she was unsure if she should attempt to reach out to this doctor for more information.

Discussion Questions

1. What should the team research to assist them in deciding about eligibility for a 504 plan? (**D10**)

2. Read the Frequently Asked Questions (FAQs) page of information from the U.S. Department of Education related to 504 plans (United States Department of Education, 2020a). Also, read their general guidance on 504 plans (United States Department of Education, 2020b). What information can be gleaned by this?
3. What are the main "takeaways" from these resources from the US Department of Education as it relates to this case? (**D10**)
4. Should Jessica qualify for a 504 Plan? Why or why not? (**D10**)
5. If she does not qualify for a 504 Plan, what other services or supports should the school be providing for Jessica? What are her needs that may not have been met by the school during her transition back to school for fifth grade? (**D3, D4**)
6. Jessica's mother is not comfortable that the school is truly understanding her concerns. Why might this be? What can the team do differently/better to develop a more collaborative relationship with Jessica's mother? (**D7**)
7. The school psychologist is interested in learning more from Jessica's oncologist. What steps should the school psychologist take to initiate this contact? Why is this potentially a critical step in determining how the school can better serve Jessica? (**D7, D10**)

Advanced Applications

1. Jessica's mother reports in the meeting about the oncologist's information regarding the potential impact of treatment for leukemia on functioning and development. Conduct research about how various treatments might impact cognitive, academic, behavioral, social, or emotional development. Report back to the group/class about these potential impacts and how this should inform how schools provide services for children with chronic health problems. (**D3, D4**)
2. What might be included in the 504 plan for Jessica? Find a 504 plan template and complete a sample plan that could be used to provide accommodations for Jessica. (**D3, D4, D10**)
3. Role play a team meeting with Jessica's parents and teachers to practice team facilitation, active listening, paraphrasing, and reflection of feelings. (**D2, D7**)
4. Review Glaser and Shaw's (2014) "Best Practices in Collaborating With Medical Personnel" chapter and Riccio et al.'s (2014) "Best Practices in

Meeting the Needs of Children With Chronic Illness." Summarize the salient points from these chapters and apply these practices to this case. (**D2, D3, D4, D7**)

References

American Psychological Association. (2017a). *Multicultural guidelines: An ecological approach to context, identity, and intersectionality.* www.apa.org/about/policy/multicultural-guidelines

American Psychological Association. (2017b). *Ethical principles of psychologists and code of conduct* (2002, amended effective June 1, 2010, and January 1, 2017). www.apa.org/ethics/code/

Beebe-Frankenberger, M., & Goforth, A. N. (2014). Best practices in providing school psychological services in rural settings. In P. L. Harrison & A. Thomas (Eds.), *Best practices in school psychology* (pp. 143–156). National Association of School Psychologists.

Family Educational Rights and Privacy Act of 1974, 20 U. S. C. §1232g. (1974).

Glaser, S. E., & Shaw, S. R. (2014). Best practices in collaborating with medical personnel. In P. L. Harrison & A. Thomas (Eds.), *Best practices in school psychology* (pp. 375–388). National Association of School Psychologists.

Harris, S. E., & Robinson Kurpius, S. E. (2014). Social networking and professional ethics: Client searches, informed consent, and disclosure. *Professional Psychology: Research and Practice, 45*(1), 11–19. https://doi.org/10.1037/a0033478

Individuals with Disabilities Education Improvement Act of 2004, Pub. L. No. 108–446. (2004).

Liang, B., Chung, A., Diamonti, A. J., Douyon, C. M., Gordon, J. R., Joyner, E. D., Meerkins, T. M., Rene, K. M., Sienkiewicz, S-A., Weber, A., White, A. F., & Wilson, E. S. (2017). Ethical social justice: Do the ends justify the means? *Journal of Community and Applied School Psychology, 27*(4), 298–311. https://doi.org/10.1002/casp.23233

National Association of School Psychology. (2020). *The professional standards of the national association of school psychologists.* National Association of School Psychologists.

Riccio, C. A., Beathard, J., & Rae, W. A. (2014). Best practices in meeting the needs of children with chronic illness. In P. L. Harrison & A. Thomas (Eds.), *Best practices in school psychology* (pp. 389–404). National Association of School Psychologists.

Skalski, A. K., & Myers, M. A. (2014). Best practices in the professional evaluation of school psychologists using the NASP practice model. In P. L. Harrison & A. Thomas (Eds.), *Best practices in school psychology* (pp. 599–610). National Association of School Psychologists.

United States Department of Education. (2020a, January 10). *Frequently asked questions.* https://www2.ed.gov/about/offices/list/ocr/faqs.html

United States Department of Education. (2020b, November 20). *Office for civil rights* https://www2.ed.gov/about/offices/list/ocr/index.html

Williams, B. B., & Armistead, L., & Jacob, S. (2008). *Professional ethics for school psychologists: A problem-solving model casebook.* National Association of School Psychologists.

Index

Made in the USA
Middletown, DE
30 June 2024

56620738R00110